Handbook of Transfusion Medicine

Blood Transfusion Services
of the United Kingdom
SECOND EDITION 1996

Editor: Brian McClelland

Kindly Donated

by

Dr Lund

London: HMSO

Published by HMSO and available from:

HMSO Publications Centre
(Mail, fax and telephone orders only)
PO Box 276, London SW8 5DT
Telephone orders 0171-873 9090
General enquiries 0171-873 0011
(queuing system in operation for both numbers)
Fax orders 0171-873 8200

HMSO Bookshops
49 High Holborn, London WC1V 6HB
0171-873 0011 Fax 0171-831 1326 (counter service only)
68-69 Bull Street, Birmingham B4 6AD
0121-236 9696 Fax 0121-236 9699
33 Wine Street, Bristol BS1 2BQ
0117-926 4306 Fax 0117 9294515
9-21 Princess Street, Manchester M60 8AS
0161-834 7201 Fax 0161-833 0634
16 Arthur Street, Belfast BT1 4GD
01232 238451 Fax 01232 235401
71 Lothian Road, Edinburgh EH3 9AZ
0131-228 4181 Fax 0131-229 2734
The HMSO Oriel Bookshop,
The Friary, Cardiff CF1 4AA
01222 395548 Fax 01222 384347

The Parliamentary Bookshop
12 Bridge Street, Parliament Square,
London SW1A 2JX
Telephone orders 0171-219 3890
General enquiries 0171-219 3890
Fax orders 0171-219 3866

HMSO's Accredited Agents
(see Yellow Pages)

and through good booksellers

Contents

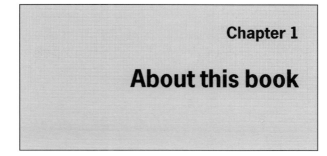

Chapter 1

About this book

About this book

Audience

This book is for staff who are responsible for prescribing, supplying and administering blood products. Many people have an essential part in making sure that the right blood product is given to the right patient at the right time. They include:

- Medical staff who assess the patient and prescribe and order the product.
- Laboratory staff who receive the order and prepare the product, matching it to the patient's blood group where necessary.
- Transport and delivery personnel who deliver the product to the patient.
- Nurses, who have a critically important responsibility in carrying out the checks before the product is administered and observing the patient during and after the transfusion.

Evidence

Correctly used, blood and blood products can save lives and provide clinical benefit to many patients. However, the effectiveness of much of today's blood transfusion practice has not been rigorously proved by clinical trials. It is therefore not possible to give a complete, evidence based guideline for practice. We have tried to use existing evidence about effective treatment. Where good evidence is not available, the contents reflect our best effort to give a balanced view of current opinion about good clinical practice in transfusion for patients in the United Kingdom.

It is important to emphasise that in other parts of the world, decisions about safe and effective practice have to take account of different local situations, for example epidemiology of infectious diseases, availability of intravenous fluids, and access to supplies of good quality blood products.

Key topics

Most of the problems with transfusion that cause delays and may put the patient at risk are caused by poor communication or failure to follow procedures that should be well documented and in which staff should be well trained. Common problems include:

- Prescribing blood products that are not required by the patient or are not the most suitable for the patient's needs.
- Incomplete or inaccurate completion of request forms or sample tube labels.
- Delays caused by a failure to communicate accurately when and where the blood is needed.
- Transfusion of blood products that were intended to be given to someone else.
- Failure to recognise and react effectively to evidence of adverse reactions that occur during transfusion.

Some rare complications of transfusion, such as the transmission of viral, infections, may only be recognisable many days or weeks after the blood product has been given. Clinical staff have the responsibility of recognising and reporting problems of this type to the supplier (usually the hospital transfusion department [HTD]). It is the task of the producer (the Blood Transfusion Service or other manufacturer of the blood product) to ensure that the products supplied are as safe and as effective as possible and that reported adverse events are effectively followed up.

Glossary of terms and abbreviations

Apheresis (Single Donor) Platelet Concentrate	Platelets prepared by apheresis of the donor
Apheresis (Single Donor) Plasma	Plasma prepared by apheresis of the donor
Artificial Colloid Solutions	Gelatins, dextrans, hydroxyethyl starch
Anti-D Immunoglobulin	Human IgG preparation containing a high level of antibody to the Rh D antigen

Autologous Transfusion	General term for several techniques e.g. – preoperative blood donation – perioperative isovolaemic haemodilution – salvage from operation site (intraoperative) – salvage from operation site (postoperative)
BCSH	British Committee for Standards in Haematology
Blood Components	Whole blood, red cells, plasma, platelets, cryoprecipitate prepared in the Regional Transfusion Centre
Blood Products	Any therapeutic product derived from human whole blood or plasma donations
CABG	Coronary artery bypass grafting
Colloid Solutions (Artificial Colloids)	Gelatin; Dextran, starch preparations: table 12 page 51.
CMV	Cytomegalovirus
Crystalloid Solutions	Saline, Ringer's lactate etc.
DAGT	Direct antiglobulin test (Coombs' test) - sensitive method to detect red cell bound antibody
DIC	Disseminated intravascular coagulation
Epoietin	Approved name for recombinant human erythropoietin
EPO	Abbreviation for erythropoietin
FFP	Fresh frozen plasma. Plasma that is frozen within a specific time period after collection and stored in the frozen state until thawed for transfusion or crushed for fractionation.
GvHD	Graft versus host disease
HAV	Hepatitis A virus
HBV	Hepatitis B virus
HCV	Hepatitis C virus
HTLV	Human T Cell Leukaemia virus

Human Parvovirus B19	A non-enveloped virus transmissible by blood products and potentially pathogenic in some groups of patients
INR	International normalised ratio: a standardised way of expressing prothrombin time ratio for monitoring of coumarin anticoagulation
Kleihauer Test	Acid elution of blood film to allow counting of fetal cells in maternal blood
Massive Transfusion	Transfusion in acute haemorrhage often defined as replacement of 1 blood volume within 24 hours
MVB	Microvascular bleeding: Bleeding from mucous membrane; oozing from catheter sites which persists after application of pressure; continuous oozing from surgical wound and raw tissue surfaces; generalised petechiae or increased size of ecchymoses.
NANB Hepatitis	Non A Non B hepatitis: former operational term for the most common class of post-transfusion hepatitis. Now known to be largely due to Hepatitis C virus and >80% eliminated by HCV screening of donations.
PCC	Prothrombin complex concentrate
Plasma Fractions	Partially or highly purified human plasma proteins prepared under pharmaceutical manufacturing conditions and generally licensed by MCA
PTH	Post-transfusion hepatitis
PTR	Prothrombin time ratio (see also INR)
Recovered Plasma	Plasma prepared from individual donations of whole blood
Recovered (Random Donor) Platelet Concentrate	Platelets prepared from individual donations of whole blood
Red Cells	The term is used for any red cell component unless otherwise stated
Rh D	The most immunogenic antigen of the Rhesus blood group system

Saline	Sodium chloride intravenous infusion 0.9%
TPH	Transplacental haemorrhage
TTP	Thrombotic thrombocytopenic purpura
Viral Inactivation	Additional manufacturing step in making blood products: validated to remove or substantially reduce infectivity for specified viruses. Some viruses may not be reliably inactivated by all the current methods.

Feedback

This second edition of the handbook has been improved by many comments and criticisms received from users of the first edition. The production team depend on readers of this edition to help improve the next revision.

Please E-Mail your comments, ideas and criticisms to the editor Brian McClelland@SNBTS1.SNBTS.SCOT.NHS.UK. or FAX to 44 (0)131-53-65352.

Authorship

The people who prepared and evaluated this handbook are listed below. If you need specialist advice, you may find it useful to contact one of them. We will do our best to give an answer to your questions – and to include the important points in the next edition of the handbook.

Editor:

D B L McClelland
Director, Edinburgh & South East Scotland Blood Transfusion Service
41 Lauriston Place
Edinburgh EH3 9HB

Contributors:

J A J Barbara
Consultant in Microbiology to the
National Blood Service, England
North London Blood
Transfusion Centre
Colindale Avenue
London NW9 5BG

M Brennan
Consultant
North London Blood
Transfusion Centre
Colindale Avenue
London NW9 5BG

S C Davies
Consultant
Central Middlesex Hospital
Acton Lane
Park Royal
London NW10 7NS

J Gillon
Consultant, Edinburgh & South East
Scotland Blood Transfusion Service
41 Lauriston Place
Edinburgh EH3 9HB

S M Knowles
Consultant and Clinical Director
South Thames Blood Transfusion
Service
75 Cranmer Terrace
Tooting
London SW17 0RB

W G Murphy
Senior Lecturer, University of
Edinburgh Medical School
41 Lauriston Place
Edinburgh EH3 9HB

J A F Napier
Consultant and Medical Director
National Blood Transfusion Service
(Wales)
Rhydlafar
St. Fagans
Cardiff CF5 6XF

W H Ouwehand
Lecturer
Division of Transfusion Medicine
University of Cambridge
East Anglian Blood Centre
Long Road
Cambridge CB2 2PT

R R C Stewart
Formerly, Product Services Manager
Scottish National Blood Transfusion
Service
Now at, Inveresk
Clinical Research Ltd.
Research Park
Heriot Watt University
Riccarton
Edinburgh EH14

A Todd
Consultant
Edinburgh & South East Scotland
Blood Transfusion Service
41 Lauriston Place
Edinburgh EH3 9HB

L M Williamson
Lecturer
Division of Transfusion Medicine
University of Cambridge
East Anglian Blood Centre
Long Road
Cambridge CB2 2PT

P L Yap
Consultant, Edinburgh & South East
Scotland Blood Transfusion Service
41 Lauriston Place
Edinburgh EH3 9HB

Reviewers

F Ala
Director
West Midlands Regional Blood
Transfusion Centre
Vincent Drive
Edgbaston
Birmingham B15 2SG

J D Cash
Medical & Scientific Director
Scottish National Blood Transfusion
Service
Ellen's Glen Road
Edinburgh EH17 7QT

M Contreras
Chief Executive and Medical Director
North London Blood Transfusion
Centre
Colindale Avenue
London NW9 5BG

M Greaves
Consultant
Department of Haematology
Royal Hallamshire Hospital
Glossop Road
Sheffield S10 2JF

F Hill
Consultant
Department of Haematology
The Children's Hospital
Ladywood Middleway
Ladywood
Birmingham B16 8ET

J S Lilleyman
Professor of Paediatric Oncology
St. Bartholomew's Hospital
London EC1A 7BE

A H Waters
Department of Haematology
St. Batholomew's Hospital
West Smithfield
London EC1A 7BE

JK Wood
Consultant
Department of Haematology
The Leicester Royal Infirmary
Leicester LE1 5WW

Acknowledgement

The manuscript was prepared for publication by Mrs Irene McKechnie, Edinburgh & South East Scotland Blood Transfusion Service. The figures were prepared by Mr Michael McLaughlin and Mr Robert Clarkson, ESEBTS.

We thank many other colleagues who have commented on the text and assisted with references.

Local systems and procedures

If you are not familiar with the local system for obtaining blood products, visit the blood bank. The clinical and technical staff there will be able to explain the system. There is no substitute for talking with the people who are working to help you care for your patients.

Blood ordering in an emergency

Procedures for identification of the patient and labelling of tubes and forms must be strictly followed.

The blood bank should be informed as quickly as possible of the quantity of blood needed and the time it is needed. Special transport arrangements may be required.

In some situations the blood bank may advise the use of Group O blood, but usual practice in the UK is to provide blood of the patient's ABO and Rh D group. This can usually be issued within 15 minutes of the blood bank receiving a patient's blood sample. Local arrangements vary. **If your job is likely to involve urgent blood ordering you must make yourself familiar with the local system.**

Unmatched Group O blood should only be requested and used when the patient's life would be at risk if there were any delay in giving blood. Group O negative blood is almost always in short supply. If it is used when it is not absolutely necessary, the supply for other real emergencies will be depleted.

Figure 1:   The blood transfusion process from donors to patients

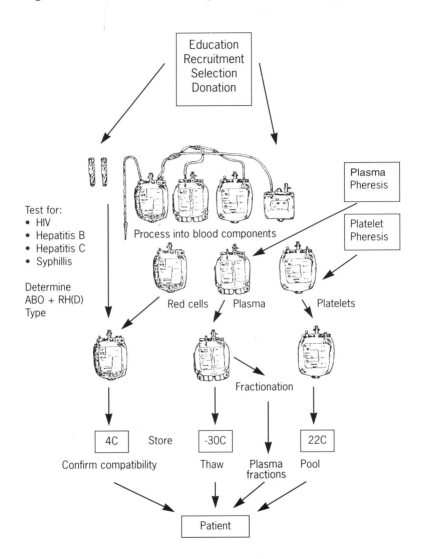

Names of blood products

In this book we have used the following convention.

– *Blood products*	Any therapeutic substances prepared from human blood.
– *Blood components*	Red cells Fresh frozen plasma Platelets Cryoprecipitate White cells Progenitor cells collected from peripheral blood (stem cells).
– *Plasma fractions*	These are partially purified human plasma proteins made under pharmaceutical manufacturing conditions, including coagulation factors, immunoglobulins and albumin.

Names of other fluids

The following short terms are used in the text.

– *Crystalloid*	Saline, Dextrose, Ringer's solution, etc.
– *Saline*	Sodium chloride injection 0.9% BP.
– *Colloids*	Dextran, modified fluid gelatin, hydroxyethyl starch *(see BNF for details)*.

The concept of blood component therapy

It is useful for the prescriber to understand a few basic facts about how blood is collected and processed because this affects the safety and availability of the products. *Figure 1* illustrates the processing of blood from donor to patient. Blood is a raw material from which a range of therapeutic products including platelet concentrate, red cells and fresh frozen plasma are made. Large amounts of plasma are also needed for the production of plasma fractions such as albumin, coagulation factors and immunoglobulins. In the United Kingdom most of the plasma is obtained from whole blood donations as shown in the figure. Some is obtained by plasmapheresis.

Blood donors and blood donation testing

Donors can give 450 ml whole blood, generally up to 3 times per year. Donors up to 60 yrs may alternatively give up to 15 litres of plasma per year by plasmapheresis: each donation provides 500-600 ml of plasma. Platelets and leucocytes can also be collected by cytapheresis.

The medical selection of donors is intended to exclude anyone whose blood might harm the recipient, for example by transmitting infection. In the UK every blood donation is tested for evidence of infection with Hepatitis B, Hepatitis C, HIV-1, HIV-2 and Syphilis. In other countries, different tests for infection may also be needed, depending on the frequency of infection in the community. Each donation is tested to determine the blood group (ABO and Rh D).

Table 1: *Blood donors and donation*

- **Healthy persons aged 18-65 can give blood***

  At each attendance donors complete a questionnaire or are interviewed to identify those

  – who could be harmed by donating

  – whose blood could harm a patient

- **Donation may be**

  – Whole blood: 2-3 times per year

  – Plasma by apheresis: up to 15 per year

  – Platelets by apheresis: up to 24 times per year

Blood donations from relatives or friends (directed donation)

Blood provided by a patient's relatives or friends specifically for that patient is called 'directed' donation. This does not reduce the risk of virus transmission. Directed donations may on occasion be less safe since the donors may not be true volunteers and may have reasons for being reluctant to disclose information that should exclude them from donation.

There are occasional circumstances, such as neonatal alloimmune thrombocytopenia in which it may be necessary to transfuse a mother's platelets to her baby. Other types of directed donation should be discouraged.

Irradiation
Donations from blood relatives can cause fatal graft versus host disease. Therefore if a patient has to receive blood from a relative, any cellular blood component *must* be irradiated.

* 17-70 in Scotland

Preparation of blood components

Blood is collected into sterile plastic packs which are centrifuged to separate red cells, platelets and plasma (Figure 1). Plasma prepared in this way or obtained by plasmapheresis may be further processed into plasma fractions.

Manufacture of plasma fractions

Plasma fractions are partially purified therapeutic preparations of plasma proteins. They are manufactured in a large scale pharmaceutical process from large volumes of plasma. Typically the plasma from up to 20,000 individual donations, about 5,000 kg of plasma, is processed by the addition of ethanol and exposure to varying temperature, pH and ionic strength conditions to precipitate different proteins. Further purification and virus inactivation steps are carried out. The final products are freeze dried powders or solutions.

Since plasma from any one of the individual donors who contribute to each batch of products could potentially introduce infectious organisms, careful screening of every donation is vital. Even with screening, some viruses could find their way into the pooled plasma, so the manufacturing processes include steps to inactivate any infectious agents which might escape detection.

Labels

Blood components carry labels applied by the Blood Centre that produced them and also by the hospital transfusion department. The Blood Centre labels contain the information that is important for staff who administer products and also allow the origins of the product to be traced. The label applied by the hospital transfusion department should contain information that uniquely identifies the patient for whom the component has been selected. *An essential step before administering any blood component is to make sure that the details on this label (usually called the 'compatibility label') match exactly with the identity of the patient (page 37). Figure 2 shows the main features of blood component labels.*

Figure 2: Blood component label: The example shown is for red cells in additive solution. Important information is shown in barcode as well as conventional characters to help computerised data entry.

Name of manufacturer, product licence number, type of plastic

Donation number

Expiry date ("use before")

Correct testing, storage and administration of blood components make transfusion very safe but this cautionary note is a reminder that zero risk cannot be guaranteed

Blood group and Rhesus D type of red cells

Collection centre

Details of blood pack: lot and type

Chapter 2

Blood products

Blood products

Essential Information

The tables that follow summarise important information about the use, storage and content of blood products. More information is available in the 'further reading' section, or from your supplier of blood products.

Table 2: *Blood products – virological safety*

- All donations of whole blood, plasma and platelets are tested to exclude the following viruses transmissible by blood: Hepatitis B, Hepatitis C, HIV 1 and 2
- Blood components are not routinely subjected to further manufacturing procedures to reduce risk of virus transmission
- The exceptions are:
  Virus inactivated plasma
  Leucocyte filtered components (effective leucocyte filtration removes the risk of transmitting cytomegalovirus)
  CMV antibody negative components (exclusion of components containing antibody removes the risk of transmitting CMV)
- Plasma Fractions are subjected to further manufacturing procedures to remove or reduce the risk of transmission of Hepatitis B, Hepatitis C, HIV and other viruses

---

Table 3: *Blood components – storage and administration*

	Red Cells Red cells (Additive) Whole Blood	Platelet Concentrate Recovered (Random Donor)	Platelet Concentrate Apheresis (Single Donor)	Fresh Frozen Plasma	Cryoprecipitate
Storage temperature	2 to 6C	At 20–24C on a special agitator rack		−30C	−30C
Shelf life	35 days	5 days	5 days	1 year (frozen)	1 year (frozen)
Longest time from leaving controlled storage to completing infusion	5 hours	Depends on preparation method: consult supplier		4 hours after thawing	4 hours after thawing
Compatibility testing requirement	Must be compatible with recipient's ABO and Rh D type and clinically significant red cell antibodies	Preferably ABO compatible. Rhesus negative females under the age of 45 years should be given Rh D negative platelets	Should be ABO compatible to avoid risk of haemolysis caused by donor Anti A or Anti B		

Points to Note:
Administration
- Infuse through a blood administration set
- Record details of each blood component infusion in the patient's case record
- Follow local procedures or protocols for ordering and administering blood components

Table 4: *Red cell products*

Unit	Red Cells	Red Cells, Additive Solution**	Red Cells, Buffy Coat Removed	Red Cells, Leucocyte Depleted	Whole Blood
Unit			1 Donation		
*Volume ml	280 ± 60	350 ± 70	280 ± 60	280 ± 60	450 ± 45
Haematocrit %	0.55 – 0.75	0.50 – 0.70	0.50 – 0.70	0.50 – 0.75	0.35 – 0.45
Packed Red Cells ml per unit			120 – 250		
White Cells per unit			$<1.2 \times 10^{9}$	$<5 \times 10^{6}$	
Content per unit *Sodium mmol Fresh* Expiry	15 / 10	20 / 15	As for starting component.		50 / 55
*Potassium mmol Fresh Expiry	0.3 / 6	0.5 / 5			1 / 9
*Lactate mmol Fresh Expiry			1 / 10		
*Hydrogen ion nmol Fresh Expiry	5 / 12				20 / 55

Table 4: *Red cell products continued*

	Red Cells	Red Cells, Additive Solution**	Red Cells, Buffy Coat Removed	Red Cells, Leucocyte Depleted	Whole Blood
Added Chemicals**	**Citrate Phosphate Dextrose Adenine (CPDA)**	**Adenine Mannitol Glucose Sodium Chloride (SAGM)**	**CPDA or SAGM**	**CPDA or SAGM**	**CPDA**
Points to Note:		Not recommended for exchange or large volume transfusion of neonates	May reduce the risk of non haemolytic febrile transfusion reactions in patients who have reacted to previous transfusion	Can help to reduce the development of allo-antibodies to leucocyte antigens. An alternative to CMV negative product. Should NOT be used to avoid risk of GvHD: for this indication *irradiated components MUST be used*	The large volume of plasma increases risk of hypervolaemia and cardiac failure in susceptible patients

A dose of 4 ml/Kg raises venous Hb by about 1g/dl

* Typical values are given. Full product specifications are in the 'Red Guide' and SNBTS Compendium [see Further reading]

** Additive solutions are used to resuspend packed red cells after plasma is removed. They are designed to maintain the red cells in good condition during storate. There are various formulas. A widely used additive solution contains saline, adenine, glucose and mannitol (SAGM).

Table 5: *Platelet products*

	Platelets Recovered (Random Donor)	Leucocyte Depleted Apheresis Platelets	Apheresis (Single Donor) Platelets	HLA Compatible Apheresis Platelets	Crossmatched Apheresis Platelets
Unit			← 1 Donation →		
*Volume	40-60 ml of plasma per donation		← Check local product specification →		
Content of platelets	At least 55 × 10⁹ per donation		← >240 × 10⁹ →		
Content of white cells	<0.2 × 10⁹/donation	<5 × 10⁶	← <0.8 ×10⁹ →		
Points to Note Prescribing		Can help to reduce development of allo-antibodies to leucocyte antigens. An alternative to CMV-negative product		Donors are selected to match recipient for some HLA antigens May be effective in patients who do not respond to platelets due to HLA antibodies	Donors are selected by a test for reaction with recipient's plasma May be effective in patients who do not respond to platelets due to HLA antibodies
	Adult dose 4-6 donations containing >240 × 10⁹ platelets	**Contain sufficient volume of a single donor's plasma, to cause a risk of haemolysis if the donor has potent red cell antibodies. Donor should be ABO compatible** ← Adult dose: 1 donation →			

*Typical volumes are given.

Table 6: *Fresh frozen plasma and cryoprecipitate*

	Recovered (Random Donor) FFP	Apheresis (Single Donor) FFP	Cryosupernatant Plasma	Cryoprecipitate
Unit	← 1 Donation →			
Volume ml	150–300 plasma containing anticoagulant solution	500–600 of plasma containing anticoagulant solution	150–250	10–20
	← **Check local product specification** →			
Content per 200 ml Unit				
Sodium mmol			35	
Glucose mmol			4	
Potassium mmol			1	
Citrate mmol			4	
Lactate mmol			1	
Hydrogen ion nmol			12	
Fibrinogen	2–5 mg/ml	2–5 mg/ml	Low	150–300 mg/pack
von Willebrand Factor			Low	80–120 u/pack
Factor VIIIc	0.7 unit/ml	0.7 unit/ml	Low	80–120 u/pack
Other plasma proteins	← **As in slightly diluted plasma** →			
Added chemicals	← **Citrate Phosphate Dextrose Adenine** →			

Table 6: *Fresh frozen plasma and cryoprecipitate continued*

	Recovered (Random Donor) FFP	Apheresis (Single Donor) FFP	Cryo Supernatant Plasma	Cryoprecipitate
Points to Note Prescribing	• **Risk of volume overload** • **Occasional severe anaphylactic reactions, especially with rapid infusion rates** • **Infection risks are similar to those of other blood components** • **Contain normal levels of plasma immunoglobulins: including red cell antibodies that can damage recipients' red cells** • **The dosage of FFP depends upon the clinical situation and underlying disorder but 12–15 ml/kg is a generally accepted starting dose. It is important to monitor the response both clinically and with measurement of prothrombin time (PT), partial thromboplastin time (PTT) or specific factor assays**			Use virus inactivated products in preference whenever it is possible

Table 7: *Human plasma fractions*

	Human Albumin	Human Immunoglobulin	
		For intramuscular Use	*For Intravenous Use*
Unit	Typically 20g as 400 ml of 5% solution or 100 ml of 20% solution*	Varies with product and supplier	
Active constituents include	Human albumin	Human IgG –from a large pool of unselected donors –or from donors with high levels of anti Rh D or anti-viral antibodies	Human IgG –from a large pool of unselected donors
Other constituents include	Sodium 130–150 mmol/l Other plasma proteins Stabilizer (sodium caprylate)	Other immunoglobulins and other plasma proteins	Other immuno- globulins and other plasma proteins. Sucrose, pepsin
Main clinical uses	Hypoproteinaemic oedema with nephrotic syndrome (20%) Ascites in chronic liver disease (20%) Acute volume replacement (5%)	Prophylaxis of specific virus infections such as hepatitis A, B, Varicella Zoster. Prevention of Anti Rh (D) antibodies in at risk mothers	Treatment of inherited and acquired deficiencies of antibody formation. Treatment of immunological disorders such as auto-immune thrombocytopenic purpura (AITP)
Points to Note: Prescribing	20% solution: hyperoncotic and expands plasma volume by more than the amount infused. 5% solution: use carefully if patient is at risk of sodium retention. For acute volume replacement, there is no evidence that 5% Albumin is superior to alternative fluids.	**See page 70**	
Storage	At room temperature		

Clotting Factor Concentrates			
Factor VIII	*Factor IX*	*Prothrombin Complex Concentrate*	*Others Include*
Typically 250–500 iu in each vial			Factor VII Antithrombin III Fibrin Sealant [Recombinant Factor VIII] [Recombinant Factor VIIa] FEIBA (Factor VIII inhibitor bypassing activity concentrate)
Factor VIII	Factor IX	Factors II, IX, X. Some products contain Factor VII	
◄————— **Other human plasma proteins** —————►			See supplier's information
Treatment of haemophilia A	Treatment of haemophilia B	Replacement of multiple clotting factor deficiencies. Rapid correction of oral anti-coagulant effect	See supplier's information

See Page 61

All these products should be used under the guidance of a specialist clinician

Usually at 4C but check manufacturers' information

Blood products

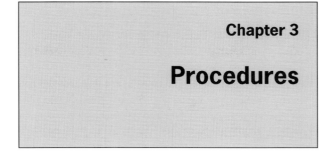

Chapter 3

Procedures

Procedures

Information for patients

Explain the proposed transfusion treatment to the patient or relatives and record in the case-notes that you have done so.

Patients or their relatives may be worried about the risks of transfusion. Some may wish to know more about the risks, about the need for transfusion and about alternatives such as autologous transfusion or drugs such as epoietin. Patients of the Jehovah's Witness faith are strictly banned by their religious beliefs from receiving blood components but may be prepared to accept plasma fractions or alternative treatments.

Research has shown that patients often have no recollection of being informed about treatment options, or feel that they have not had answers to questions that worry them. The balance of legal opinion is that a written record that the patient has been given information and that his or her questions have been answered is more valuable in a medicolegal case than the patient's signature on a consent form.

Answers to most patients' questions should be found in this book. We have also included an outline of an information sheet for patients on page 102. You should check if your hospital has a leaflet of this type and that your patients receive it.

Recording the reason for transfusion

Before blood products are administered, the reason for transfusion (which should usually comply with local or national guidelines) should be written in the patient's case-notes. This is important. If the patient later has a problem which could be related to transfusion, the records should show *who* ordered the products and *why*.

Ordering red cell products

This section may seem to be very pedantic but experience everywhere shows that **dangerous or fatal transfusion errors are usually caused by failing to keep to the standard procedures.**

Acute **haemolytic** transfusion reactions are usually caused by transfusing red cells that are incompatible with the patient's ABO type. These reactions can be fatal. They usually result from errors made in identifying the patient when samples are being taken or when blood is being administered.

When ordering and giving blood products it is therefore essential to *follow the local procedures*. These should cover the steps outlined in Figure 3.

Procedures

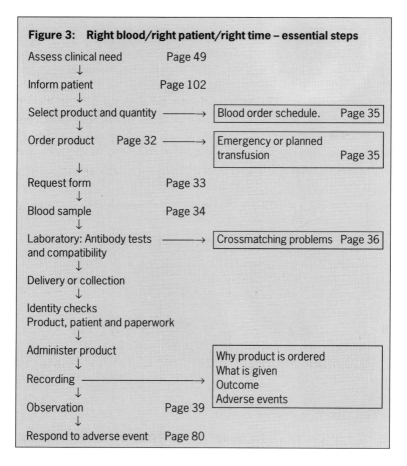

Figure 3: Right blood/right patient/right time – essential steps

Assess clinical need — Page 49
↓
Inform patient — Page 102
↓
Select product and quantity ——→ Blood order schedule. Page 35
↓
Order product — Page 32 ——→ Emergency or planned transfusion — Page 35
↓
Request form — Page 33
↓
Blood sample — Page 34
↓
Laboratory: Antibody tests and compatibility ——→ Crossmatching problems — Page 36
↓
Delivery or collection
↓
Identity checks
Product, patient and paperwork
↓
Administer product
↓
Recording ——→ Why product is ordered / What is given / Outcome / Adverse events
↓
Observation — Page 39
↓
Respond to adverse event — Page 80

Ordering blood in an emergency

This will often be done in the emergency admissions unit. There may be several unconscious patients who need blood quickly. Often many staff are involved. It is very easy to make mistakes, so *procedures must be clear and simple and everyone must know them.*

- For each patient the crossmatch sample tube and the blood request form must be clearly labelled with the EMERGENCY ADMISSION NUMBER. Use the patient's name only if you are sure you have correct information.

- If you have to send another request for the same patient within a short period, use the same identifiers that you used on the first request so the hospital transfusion department staff know they are dealing with the same patient.

- It may help if one person takes charge of ordering blood especially if several patients are involved at the same time; that person should communicate with the hospital transfusion department.

- Tell the hospital transfusion department how quickly the blood is needed for each patient. This allows the laboratory to prioritise the requests.

- Make sure that both you and the hospital transfusion department staff know
  - *who* is going to bring the blood to the patient
  - *where* the patient will be. For example if your patient is just about to be transferred for a CAT scan in another part of the hospital, make sure the blood will be delivered to the CAT scan room.

- The hospital transfusion department may send Group O Rhesus negative blood, especially if there is a risk of mistakes in patient identification. During an acute emergency, this may be the safest way to avoid a mismatched transfusion.

Prescribing blood products

It is the doctor's responsibility to prescribe blood products specifying the quantity to be given, duration of infusion and any other special precautions.

Request forms for compatibility testing

- The blood request form should be clearly and accurately completed with the patient's family name, given name, date of birth and hospital number.

- Patients who at the time of admission cannot be reliably identified *must* be given an identity band with a unique number. This number *must* be used to identify this patient until full and correct details are available and are properly communicated to the hospital transfusion department.

- The quantity of the blood component required and the time at which it is needed should be written on the request form. The timing of blood ordering for planned procedures should comply with local rules and the quantity requested for elective surgical patients should be guided by the local surgical blood ordering schedule.
- All the details requested on the form should be completed. It should be signed by the clinician with his or her name in *legible* capitals.

Blood samples for compatibility testing

- At the time of taking the sample the conscious patient must be asked to state his or her given name, family name and date of birth.
- This information must be checked against the patient's identification bracelet to make sure that the details entered on the request form are identical.
- The blood sample should be taken according to the hospital laboratory manual and the correct sample tube must be used (for adults, usually 10 ml, no anticoagulant).
- The sample tubes must be accurately *labelled at the patient's bedside at the time the blood sample is being taken*. Sample containers must not be pre-labelled before the specimen is obtained because of the risk of putting the patient's blood into the wrong tubes.
- In the case of unconscious patients a medical practitioner should complete the request form and take the sample.

The hospital transfusion department staff are acting correctly if they refuse to accept a request for compatibility testing when either the request form or the sample is inadequately identified. At least 5% of samples arrive with labelling or form filling errors. This wastes time for all concerned and can contribute to serious errors.

In some hospitals the responsibility for taking samples from conscious patients is delegated to phlebotomists. They should be specifically trained for this work.

Blood ordering for planned procedures

Blood ordering schedule or tariff

The blood order for a planned procedure should reflect the clinical team's actual blood use for the particular operation. Many operations very rarely need transfusion so there is no need to order blood as a routine.

The type and screen procedure should be used for procedures where red cell transfusion is only rarely required.

For procedures that often need red cell transfusion, the standard blood order should be based on the actual use of blood for patients who have recently undergone that operation, not taking account of the occasional patient who has unusually severe blood loss.

Type and screen

- **Type and screen (also called 'group and hold' or 'group and save').** In the laboratory, the patient's ABO and Rh D type are determined and the patient's serum is screened for IgG antibodies that can damage red blood cells at 37C. The patient's serum sample is then held in the laboratory, usually for 7 days. If red cells are required within this period they can be provided safely for the patient after a further rapid test to exclude ABO incompatibility. Using this method the hospital transfusion department will usually need about 15 minutes to have blood ready for issue to the patient.

  With this approach there is no need to hold units of blood as an 'insurance' for a patient who is unlikely to need them. As a result we can make better use of the donated red cells.

Crossmatch

- **Red cell compatibility testing (crossmatching).** In addition to the group and screen, the patient's serum sample is usually tested by the hospital transfusion department for compatibility with the red cells of the units of blood to be transfused.*

* In some EU countries this procedure is not routine, but other checks are used instead.

Compatible units of blood are then labelled specifically for the patient and can be kept available for immediate release. The laboratory will usually reserve these units only for 48 hours after the time for which they were requested.

If the patient needs further red cell transfusion a fresh sample should be sent for crossmatching. This is especially important if more than 72 hours has elapsed since the previous cross match or if the patient has had a red cell transfusion completed more than 24 hours ago. Red cell antibodies may appear very rapidly as a result of the immunological stimulus given by transfused donor red cells.

Crossmatching problems

When the patient's sample is found to contain a clinically significant red cell antibody further tests are needed to identify the antibody so that red cell units of a suitable blood type can be provided. The laboratory may well ask for another blood sample from the patient.

Every effort will be made by the transfusion department to provide blood that is compatible to avoid the risks of haemolytic transfusion reaction or of stimulating the patient's antibody to a high level. These tests may be complicated and can cause considerable delay in providing red cells.

When this occurs, non urgent transfusions and surgery should be delayed until suitable red cell units are found, to avoid risk to the patient.

However, when a patient needs transfusion urgently and it is difficult to find compatible red cell units the doctor responsible for the transfusion department should be asked to advise on the risk of a life-threatening reaction if a red cell unit is given that is not fully compatible. *This risk must be balanced against the risk of delaying transfusion when a patient's life may be at risk from blood loss that urgently requires restoring the oxygen carrying capacity of the patient's blood.*

Storage, release and collection of red cells for transfusion

Red cells must be stored in a special, designated refrigerator. It is the responsibility of the hospital transfusion department to maintain these refrigerators and to specify the procedures to be followed when removing red cell units from them.

Crossmatched units of blood may be held within the hospital transfusion department or delivered to another blood refrigerator. In either case, the written procedure for removing red cell units for a patient should state:

- Who is authorised to collect red cell units from the refrigerator
- The details that must be checked against the labels of the units being collected
- The record that must be made of collection (and return) of the units, including:
  - the identity of the patient for whom blood is collected
  - the unique number of the red cell pack (Fig 2)
  - the time of collection
  - the name of person collecting the unit
  - the time of returning units to the refrigerator if they are not transfused

Crossmatched red cell units will be collected by the transfusion laboratory if they have not been used within 48 hours of the time for which they were originally requested. *They must be kept in the blood refrigerator except when actually being transfused.*

Administering blood products

The procedures for infusing blood components should be defined by the hospital transfusion department with the medical and nursing staff. *The written procedures should be available to all staff who have to administer transfusions.* Responsibility for ensuring that the procedures are kept up to date and available and for staff training must be defined by the hospital's management.

Identity checks

Follow local procedures for the checks to be undertaken and the staff who may perform them. The checking must involve two people, one of whom should be a Registered nurse or doctor.

The hospital transfusion department should provide with the red cell units a compatibility report stating the patient's full identity, the patient's ABO and Rh D group and the unique donation number and group of each unit which has been supplied.

The compatibility label on each unit should show:

- Family name of patient
- Given name
- Date of birth and hospital number
- Patient's ABO and Rh D group
- Unique donation number
- Date and time for which blood is requested

Occasionally red cells will be supplied that are of a different ABO group from the patient's but that are compatible – e.g. red cells of Group A are safe for a patient of Group AB. In this event (usually due to shortage of a particular group) the hospital transfusion department should inform the clinician responsible and also record the fact on the document that accompanies the blood units. Before starting the infusion check that there are NO discrepancies between:

- Information on the patient's identity band, the compatibility label and the compatibility report. Patients who can communicate should be asked to state their identity

- The ABO and Rh D group on the blood pack, on the compatibility label and in the compatibility report

- The donation number given on the blood pack, on the compatibility label and on the compatibility report

If any discrepancies are found the unit must not be transfused. If there is any suspicion that the contents of the pack appear abnormal (e.g. evidence of leakage, unusual colour or signs of haemolysis) the unit must not be transfused and the hospital transfusion department must be informed immediately.

Always check that:

- The expiry date on the blood pack has not been passed
- There is no sign of leakage from the pack

Record keeping

The person administering a blood product must enter in the casenotes the number and blood group of the unit, the type of blood component and the time at which the transfusion commenced. They must sign to indicate that the pre-administration checks have been performed. This document is part of the patient's permanent record.

Observe the patient

- Before starting the transfusion record the patient's temperature and pulse on the appropriate chart, ¼ hourly for the first half hour of each pack's administration and then hourly until completion
- When the administration is commenced record the relevant information on the Fluid Administration and Fluid Balance chart (or 24 hr chart in ITU/HDU)
- Adjust the flow-rate to achieve infusion over the prescribed time period
- Throughout the transfusion observe the patient for any sign or symptom of incompatibility or adverse reaction e.g. flushing, urticaria, vomiting, diarrhoea, fever, itching, headache, haemoglobinuria, pain at or near the transfusion site, rigor, severe backache, collapse, circulatory failure. Should any of these be observed the transfusion must be stopped immediately and the doctor informed. Keep the IV line open with a slow infusion of 0.9% Saline
- Any suspected transfusion reaction or incompatibility should be investigated according to the local procedure and advice from the hospital transfusion department.

Clinical features and management of acute transfusion reactions are on page 80.

Time limits for infusion

There is a risk of bacterial proliferation when blood components are kept at ambient temperature. For this reason a blood component transfusion must be started within 30 minutes of removing the pack from refrigeration and be completed within 5 hours of starting the transfusion. See Table 3 for other blood components.

Blood administration sets

For red cells, plasma and cryoprecipitate

Blood must be infused through a blood giving set containing an integral filter. The set must be changed at least 12 hourly during blood component infusion.

For platelets

A fresh blood administration set or platelet transfusion set, primed with saline should be used to infuse platelets.

For small children

Special paediatric sets should be used.

Filtration of red cells and platelets

Microaggregate filters

There is no evidence from controlled trials that these offer clinical benefit. Common, but unproven indications are for massively transfused patients, transfusion for multiple trauma and during cardiopulmonary bypass. Some patients who require long-term red cell replacement have febrile transfusion reactions and microaggregate filtration of stored red cells may reduce or prevent these reactions.

Leucocyte depleting filters

The technology and application of these filters is still evolving. They are useful in preventing the onset of febrile transfusion reactions in transfusion dependent patients and also in avoiding further reactions, if less costly options are not successful.

The use of effectively leucocyte depleted red cells and platelets can reduce the development of anti-leucocyte antibodies in multiple transfused patients but only if all transfused units are filtered. Many clinicians believe this delays or avoids refractoriness to platelet therapy. This remains controversial.

Blood warmers

There is no evidence that warming blood is beneficial to the patient when infusion is slow. At infusion rates greater than 100 ml/minute case reports suggest that cold blood could cause cardiac arrest. Keeping the patient warm is probably more important than warming the infused blood.

Use of a blood warmer is advised for adults receiving infusion of blood at rates greater than 50 ml/kg/hour, for children receiving volumes greater than 15 ml/kg/hour and for infants undergoing exchange transfusions. A blood warmer is also indicated when transfusing a patient who has clinically significant cold agglutinins.

Blood warmers can be dangerous if they malfunction. They must have a visible thermometer and an audible warning and be properly maintained. Red cells and plasma exposed to temperatures over 40C may cause severe transfusion reactions. Blood products must NOT be warmed by improvisations such as putting the pack into hot water, in a microwave or on a radiator.

Do not add other pharmaceuticals to blood products

No other infusion solutions or drugs should be added to any blood component. They may contain additives such as calcium which can cause citrated blood to clot. Dextrose solution (5%) can lyse red cells. Drugs should never be added to any blood product. If there is an adverse reaction it may be impossible to determine if this is due to the blood, to the medication which has been added or to an interaction of the two.

If a crystalloid or colloid solution has to be given at the same time as blood components it should normally be given through a separate IV line.

Adverse reactions

Any adverse reaction thought to be related to the transfusion should be assessed as described on page 83 and 84 and the clinical details and actions taken should be recorded in the case-notes.

Autologous transfusion

In some situations a patient can be transfused with their own blood that has been collected and stored in advance of a planned operation. This has theoretical advantages in reducing the risk of immunological incompatibility or transmission of some infectious agents. There are detailed guidelines in the UK for carrying out this procedure *(see Further reading).*

Autologous red cells can be stored for up to 5 weeks using standard hospital transfusion department conditions. Medical selection must ensure that patients are fit for this procedure. Suitable patients can donate 2-4 units of blood pre-operatively. The blood must be tested, labelled and stored to the same standard as donor blood. Before transfusion, autologous blood units must be ABO and Rh D grouped and compatibility checked to avoid the consequences of any possible clerical errors. These autologous donations should not be transfused to anyone other than the patient who provided the donation. *Do not attempt to collect autologous blood units without the advice and help of the hospital transfusion department or transfusion centre.*

There are important practical limits to the application of pre-deposit auto-transfusion.

- Not all patients are fit enough or live near enough to hospital to have 450 ml blood withdrawn several times before a planned operation

- Auto-transfusion does not reduce the risk of bacterial infection hazards that may result from collection or storage problems. Nor does it reduce the risk of procedural errors that can cause ABO incompatible transfusion

- Autologous units will often be left unused unless collection is restricted to patients undergoing operations that are very likely to involve a need for transfusion

- Some patients will need donor blood *in addition* to their autologous units

- Although pre-donation appears safe, there has been no systematic assessment of the risks

- The cost of the procedure is reported to be high in relation to the gains in patient safety

- There is new evidence that potentially dangerous mistakes occur quite frequently

Certain categories, such as young fit individuals requiring elective major surgery with inevitable blood losses are likely to benefit most from pre-deposit autologous transfusion.

Patients must be carefully informed about the procedure, especially the possibility that they may receive donor blood.

Immediate pre-operative bleeding and isovolemic haemodilution

This procedure may be useful in cardiothoracic surgery and other major procedures such as orthopaedic operations in young people. Immediately before operation, after induction of anaesthesia, blood is withdrawn with fluid replacement and stored in the operating theatre. After surgery, the patient's blood can be reinfused. This procedure allows the patient's haematocrit to be reduced to a level selected for optimal capillary perfusion, reduces red cell losses during surgery and provides fresh autologous blood for reinfusion when needed.

Intra-operative blood salvage

During surgery blood shed into the operative field can be collected by suction, mixed with anticoagulant (unnecessary if the patient is heparinised) and reinfused through a filter. Using special equipment, the red cells can be washed before reinfusion. Because of concern about the risk of contamination, cell salvage is not advised in the presence of systemic sepsis, bacterial contamination of the operation field or malignant disease.

Long term storage of autologous blood

Red cells can be stored for long periods at very low temperatures. Cryo-preservation is expensive and the facilities are available in only a few centres. It is reserved for patients with rare blood groups or with red cell antibodies that make it very difficult to find compatible donor blood.

Therapeutic apheresis

Therapeutic apheresis is the removal of blood or a blood component to benefit the patient's condition. The simplest procedure is therapeutic venesection in which whole blood (200-450 ml) is periodically withdrawn. This is indicated for some patients with haemochromatosis and polycythaemia. Alternatively cells or plasma can be selectively removed using a cell separator. Methods for selective removal of plasma constituents (e.g. cholesterol, autoantibodies) are still at the experimental stage of development.

Good venous access is essential as a rapid blood flow is required for processing. Some machines can operate using a single vein but usually separate cannulae are required for blood withdrawal and return.

Plasma exchange

Therapeutic plasma exchange combined with other medical treatment contributes effectively to management of the conditions shown in Table 8.

> **Table 8: Indications for therapeutic plasma exchange (plasmapheresis)**
>
> - Hyperviscosity syndromes e.g. myeloma, Waldenström's macroglobulinaemia
> - Rapidly progressive glomerulonephritis
> - Goodpasture's syndrome
> - Guillain-Barré syndrome
> - Familial hypercholesterolaemia
> - Thrombotic thrombocytopenic purpura

Plasma exchange has been used in many other conditions such as myasthenia gravis, pemphigus, SLE, other autoimmune disorders and in maternal Rh D sensitisation during pregnancy. Its effectiveness has not been proved in these conditions and in many cases objective monitoring is difficult. The potential risk and the high cost of plasmapheresis should be taken into account before using it in these conditions.

The replacement fluid for plasma exchange is usually 4.5% albumin, saline or a mixture of these. FFP may occasionally be needed to correct a deficiency of coagulation factors at the end of a plasma exchange.

Thrombotic thrombocytopenic purpura

This rare and serious condition often responds to infusion of fresh frozen plasma (FFP). Because of the large volumes of FFP that may have to be given, plasma exchange using FFP to replace the patient's plasma, is often used. **This is the only indication for plasma exchange with FFP.**

Cytapheresis (removal of blood cells)

Leucapheresis may help to alleviate symptoms and signs caused by very high cell counts in leukaemic patients (usually chronic granulocytic leukaemia) until chemotherapy takes effect.

Plateletpheresis is occasionally used in patients with very high platelet counts causing bleeding or thrombosis. Erythrocytapheresis is occasionally needed in the management of malaria, sickle-cell crisis, polycythaemia or following a transfusion error in which Rh D positive blood is given to a Rh D negative female of child-bearing age.

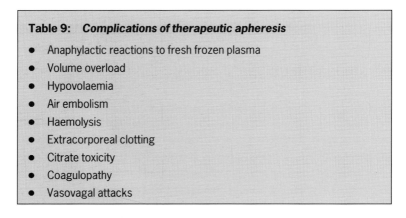

Table 9:   *Complications of therapeutic apheresis*

- Anaphylactic reactions to fresh frozen plasma
- Volume overload
- Hypovolaemia
- Air embolism
- Haemolysis
- Extracorporeal clotting
- Citrate toxicity
- Coagulopathy
- Vasovagal attacks

Progenitor cell (stem cell) collection by apheresis

Progenitor cells (autologous or allogeneic) can be collected from the peripheral blood by apheresis. This procedure is an effective alternative to the aspiration of bone marrow and avoids the need for the patient or donor to have a general anaesthetic.

This procedure must be carried out by a specialist team because the preparation of the patient, the cell collection and the laboratory procedures to process, store and prepare the patient's cells for reinfusion must be very carefully planned and coordinated. There is a detailed clinical guideline published by BCSH *(see Further reading)*

Chapter 4

Clinical applications of blood products

Clinical applications of blood products

Principles

The following section deals with clinical situations that often involve the use of one or more blood products. Some general principles that apply to most clinical decisions about transfusion are given in Table 10.

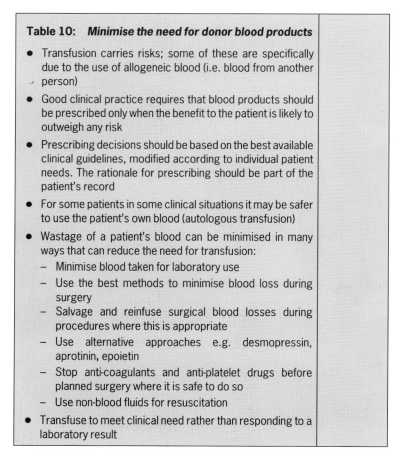

Table 10: *Minimise the need for donor blood products*

- Transfusion carries risks; some of these are specifically due to the use of allogeneic blood (i.e. blood from another person)
- Good clinical practice requires that blood products should be prescribed only when the benefit to the patient is likely to outweigh any risk
- Prescribing decisions should be based on the best available clinical guidelines, modified according to individual patient needs. The rationale for prescribing should be part of the patient's record
- For some patients in some clinical situations it may be safer to use the patient's own blood (autologous transfusion)
- Wastage of a patient's blood can be minimised in many ways that can reduce the need for transfusion:
  - Minimise blood taken for laboratory use
  - Use the best methods to minimise blood loss during surgery
  - Salvage and reinfuse surgical blood losses during procedures where this is appropriate
  - Use alternative approaches e.g. desmopressin, aprotinin, epoietin
  - Stop anti-coagulants and anti-platelet drugs before planned surgery where it is safe to do so
  - Use non-blood fluids for resuscitation
- Transfuse to meet clinical need rather than responding to a laboratory result

Perioperative red cell transfusion

When should red cell transfusion be given?

In the past surgeons and anaesthetists have often used the rule of thumb that a patient whose haemoglobin level has fallen below 10 g/dl (haematocrit <30%) needs red cell transfusion. There is no clinical evidence to support this generalisation. Some patients tolerate profound haemodilution during surgery without morbidity attributable to lack of red cells. Clinical studies do not support the general application of the '10g/30%' rule. Experimental evidence is that in healthy humans cardiac output does not increase sharply until the haemoglobin falls well below 7g/dl. However, in some older or fragile patients, especially with cardiovascular disease, even moderate haemodilution may contribute to myocardial ischaemia.

Conservative use of red cell replacement is appropriate in fit patients, especially the young who are usually very tolerant of haemodilution and for whom long term complications of avoidable transfusion are likely to be more important (Table 11).

There is however little to commend the aggressive avoidance of red cell transfusion in elderly patients. Evidence of cardiovascular and respiratory disease should lead to caution about allowing haemoglobin to fall to a low level. In all patients with substantial blood loss priority should be given to maintaining circulatory volume by giving adequate fluids and to maintaining oxygen supply.

Transfusion management of acute blood loss

This section refers to situations where rapid infusion of substantial volumes of fluid together with red cell replacement is likely to be required over a few hours as a result of major bleeding.

Clinical applications of blood products

Table 11:   *Principles of transfusion management of acute blood loss*

Insert a large IV cannula, obtain blood samples and infuse crystalloid as rapidly as possible until an acceptable systolic blood pressure is restored.

- Restore circulating fluid volume to correct hypoperfusion
- Achieve surgical control of bleeding
- Maintain adequate blood oxygen transport capacity
- Request early coagulation screen. The results may help to guide blood component therapy should bleeding persist after attempted surgical haemostasis

% Loss of Blood Volume	Equivalent Adult Fluid Volume	Replacement Fluid
<20%	Up to 1 litre	– Crystalloid (e.g. 0.9% saline)
>20%	More than 1 litre	– Red Cells – Fluid: Crystalloid and/or colloid

Notes:

1 To estimate blood volume: = 70 ml/kg in adults: 80 ml/kg in infants.

2 See Table 13, page 57 for clinical features.

3 If bleeding continues after attempted surgical haemostasis and when coagulation tests or platelet count are abnormal, platelets, FFP or cryoprecipate or combinations of these may be needed: the dose should be estimated and the effect monitored by clinical evidence of reduced bleeding, coagulation screen and platelet count.

4 Clinical trials in humans have not demonstrated that albumin solutions or colloids are superior to crystalloids for resuscitation, but much larger volumes of crystalloids are required.

5 Dextran and HES (Table 12) should be limited to 1.5 litre per 24 hours in an adult (according to manufacturers' data sheets).

6 Avoid saline in patients with severe liver disease for whom sodium overload is a special risk. Also take care with 5% Albumin in these patients for the same reason.

7 Clinical observations that should be routinely monitored and recorded throughout the management of an episode of bleeding are pulse rate, systolic BP, pulse pressure, urine output (catheter). CVP, arterial line and pulmonary artery catheter may also be required.

8 The type of crystalloid or colloid to be used and the source of supply should be specified in local protocols.

Table 12: *Non plasma colloid volume expanders*

Product	Source	Concentration of solution	Number average Mol. wt.	Intravascular persistence	Approximate frequency of severe acute reactions
Modified Fluid Gelatin	Heat-degraded cattle bone gelatin	3-4%	35,000	50% of infused volume persists 4-5 hours	1 in 10,000 infusions
Hydroxy-ethyl starch (HES)	Maize starch, chemically modified	6%	450,000 or 265,000	Similar to or longer than Dextran 70	1 in 20,000 infusions
Dextran 70	Hydrolysed starch	6%	70,000	50% of infused volume persists 24 hours	1 in 10,000 infusions
Dextran 40	Hydrolysed starch	10%	40,000	Shorter than Dextran 70	1 in 50,000 infusions

Obstetric haemorrhage

Haemorrhage remains an important cause of maternal mortality. The bleeding may be unpredicted and massive. The patient's life may depend on a fast effective response from the obstetric team, with the support of the hospital transfusion department.

There is a guideline for transfusion on obstetric bleeding in the report on 'Confidential enquiries into maternal deaths in the United Kingdom 1988-1990'. *(see Further reading).* Its main features are given on page 52.

Each obstetric unit should have a current protocol for major bleeding incidents and staff should be familiar with it.

Table 11a: *Transfusion in obstetric bleeding*

- Set up at least two I.V. lines. Use a compression cuff on the infusion pack and monitor central venous pressure (CVP) and arterial pressure. At the same time take blood for compatibility and coagulation screen. Typically a minimum of six units of red cells should be ordered.

- Summon the extra staff required, (obstetrician, midwives, nurses and anaesthetist). Alert haematologist in hospital transfusion department. Make sure porters are available at short notice.

- Fluid and red cell replacement – page 50.

- If the blood bank is informed of the urgency, ABO and Rh D compatible blood can usually be made available rapidly after receipt of the sample.

- If red cell loss is life-threatening, uncrossmatched Group O Rh-negative red cells should be used if this is the fastest available source of red cells.

- Regular haemoglobin or haematocrit assessment helps to monitor blood and fluid therapy, *but restoration of normovolaemia is the first priority*.

- Coagulation screens should be performed to help detect haemostatic failure (usually due to DIC) and to guide the use of blood components.

- Patients with major haemorrhage require effective monitoring of pulse rate, blood pressure, CVP, blood gases and acid-base status. A urinary catheter should be inserted and urine output monitored. Dedicated care by the midwifery, nursing and medical staff is vital. Transfer to ITU or HDU should be considered *early*.

Transfusion support of major bleeding problems

Acquired haemostatic problems

Haemostatic failure can be triggered by hypovolaemia, tissue damage, hypoxia or sepsis.

Normal haemostasis involves pro-coagulant proteins (the coagulation cascade), the platelets, the fibrinolytic system, and the blood vessel wall. Acquired haemostatic disorders arise frequently in hospital practice. Blood component therapy is often required. Prescribing should be based on correct interpretation of clinical features and laboratory tests.

Disseminated intravascular coagulation (DIC) refers to a spectrum of haemostatic problems. Activation of the coagulation and fibrinolytic systems leads to deficiencies of coagulation proteins, fibrinogen, and platelets. The clinical presentation can range from major bleeding with or without thrombotic complications to a compensated state detectable only on laboratory testing.

Treatment should focus on correcting the cause of DIC. Replacement with blood products is indicated when there is bleeding with acute DIC. Platelets, fresh frozen plasma, and cryoprecipitate should be given to correct thrombocytopenia and clotting factor deficiencies. Control of bleeding is the goal; laboratory test results help to select the blood products that may be effective and to monitor the doses needed.

Neonates, patients with marrow disorders or liver disease and patients taking anticoagulants, aspirin or other non steroidal anti-inflammatory drugs are more likely to develop haemostatic problems because their platelet function is impaired and/or their haemostatic factor production is reduced. Where possible, seek advice from the hospital haematology or transfusion department physicians when managing these problems.

Blood component replacement

Dilution effect

When there is no pre-existing haemostatic problem replacement of up to 1 blood volume (8-10 units of blood in an adult) with red cells and non-plasma fluids is unlikely to cause haemostatic problems due to dilution.

Platelets

In an adult, platelets should be given if there is severe microvascular bleeding (MVB) with a platelet count below 50-100 x 10^9/l, (especially if more than one blood volume has been replaced) or if laboratory results suggest there is DIC.

Clinical applications of blood products

There is no evidence that giving prophylactic platelets or plasma to patients undergoing large transfusions reduces the risk of MVB. *Routine prophylactic use of these products for major surgery is not recommended.*

Fresh frozen plasma (FFP) and cryoprecipitate

FFP should be used only where there is microvascular bleeding with laboratory results that show abnormal coagulation. A dose of 15 ml/kg is conventional (Table 6). If the fibrinogen level is below 1 g/l and DIC has been diagnosed with severe bleeding the fibrinogen level should be raised by giving cryoprecipitate (initially in an adult at least 15 packs containing in total 3-4 gm fibrinogen).

Laboratory tests of haemostasis

These can help to identify the need for blood components to control microvascular bleeding. The platelet count, prothrombin time ratio (PTR) or activated partial thromboplastin time (APTT) should be monitored during large transfusions to help guide replacement.

Other complications of large volume transfusions

The problems described below are rarely due to transfusion alone and cannot be avoided simply by attention to transfusion practice. However transfusion should be managed so as to avoid making the problems worse.

Hypocalcaemia

The citrate anticoagulant in some blood components (Table 4) binds ionised calcium. This could lower plasma ionised calcium levels, but usually rapid liver metabolism of citrate prevents this. In neonates and patients who are hypothermic, the combined effects of hypocalcaemia and hyperkalaemia may be cardiotoxic. If there is ECG or clinical evidence of hypocalcaemia, 5 ml of 10% calcium gluconate (for an adult) should be given IV. If necessary the dose should be repeated till the ECG is normal. Note that red cells in additive solution contain only traces of citrate

Hyperkalaemia

The plasma or additive solution in a unit of red cells or whole blood stored for 4-5 weeks may contain 5-10 mmol of potassium. In the presence of acidaemia and hypothermia this additional potassium can lead to cardiac arrest. This problem is best prevented by keeping the patient warm.

Hypothermia

Rapid transfusion of blood at 4C can lower the core temperature by several degrees. The best safeguard is to keep the patient warm. A blood warmer should be used in adults receiving large volumes of blood at rates above 50 ml/kg/hr (in children above 15 ml/kg/hr).

Acid base disturbances

Despite the lactic acid content of transfused blood, (1-2 mmol/unit of red cells, 3-10 mmol/unit of whole blood) fluid resuscitation usually *improves* acidosis in a shocked patient. In practice, transfused citrate can contribute to metabolic *alkalosis* when large volumes of blood components are infused.

Adult respiratory distress syndrome

The risk is minimised if good perfusion and oxygenation are maintained and over-transfusion is avoided. The use of albumin solutions to maintain a plasma oncotic pressure >20mmHg is often stated to be important but controlled studies have not proven any advantage of albumin solution over crystalloid fluids for resuscitation. The use of microaggregate filters when stored blood is transfused is often advised but the benefits remain unproven. These filters may offer benefit for patients with pre-existing lung disease (see TRALI page 88).

Avoidable haemostatic problems in the elective surgery patient

If a patient admitted for elective surgery or an invasive procedure is found to have thrombocytopenia or an abnormal coagulation screen (prolonged PTR or APPT) the procedure should be postponed while the cause of the abnormality is identified. If a congenital bleeding disorder is found, the patient must be managed in conjunction with a Haemophilia Centre.

If the platelet count is below $80 \times 10^9/l$ before starting a procedure likely to cause significant blood loss or bleeding in a critical site e.g. CNS, it must be investigated before starting the procedure.

Warfarin

Unless it is contra-indicated to do so, warfarin anticoagulation should be stopped before elective major surgery in time to allow the prothrombin time ratio to approach normal. This should be guided by a local protocol for preoperative anticoagulant management.

Aspirin

A single dose of ½ tablet, 150 mg (or ½ junior aspirin, 75 mg), impairs platelet function for several days. Aspirin should be stopped at least 7 days before planned major surgery if it is safe to do so. When an aspirin-induced platelet defect contributes to abnormal bleeding platelet transfusion is likely to be effective.

Transfusion for acute gastrointestinal bleeding

In the UK gastrointestinal bleeding occurs in 50-150/100,000 of the population each year. It is the direct cause of 3,500 deaths per year and accounts for about 8% of medical admissions to hospital.

Blood replacement for patients with GI bleeding is summarised in Table 13. Special points in managing patients with bleeding from varices associated with chronic liver disease are given in Table 14.

Table 13: *Use of fluids and blood products in managing patients with acute gastrointestinal bleeding*

Severity	Clinical Features	IV Infusion	End Point

Severe	• History of collapse and/or
	
	• Shock
	  – systolic BP <100 mmHg
	  – pulse> 100/min
		• Replace fluid rapidly page 50
		• Ensure red cells are available quickly; use local emergency transfusion protocol
		• Transfuse red cells according to clinical assessment and Hb/Hct (page 50)
			Maintain urine output >0.5 ml/kg/ hr and systolic BP >100mHg.
			Maintain haemoglobin above >9 g/dl

Significant	Resting pulse >100/min and/or haemoglobin < 10 g/dl	Replace fluid. Order compatible red cells (4 units)	Maintain haemoglobin > 9 g/dl
Trivial	Pulse and haemoglobin normal	• Maintain intravenous access until diagnosis is clear • Send patient sample for red cell group and antibody screen	

Table 14: Replacing gastrointestinal blood loss in patients with chronic liver disease

Features	Transfusion Mangement	End Points
• Bleeding is often but not always from oesophageal varices and is often severe. Other causes such as peptic ulcer are not uncommon and must be excluded	Insert one or two large bore cannulas. A central line may be indicated.	Systolic pressure >100 mmHg Haemoglobin >9 g/dl Urine output >0.5 ml/kg/hr.
• Bleeding from varices usually recurs if there is no intervention to control the varices or to reduce portal pressure. The prognosis depends on the severity of the liver disease. *	Ensure red cells are available quickly; use local emergency transfusion protocol: order 4-6 units.	CVP 0-5 mmHg (not higher)
• Hepatic failure may follow variceal bleeding, but usually recovers if bleeding can be stopped and recurrence prevented.	Crystalloids should be used carefully. Saline should be avoided as sodium retention is usual and leads to ascites.	
• Thrombocytopenia is usual. The platelet count may fall below 50 x 10⁹/l. Provided the platelet count is above 50 x 10⁹/l, bleeding is unlikely to be controlled or prevented by platelet transfusion.	Platelet transfusion is rarely needed. If there is continued bleeding with a platelet count below 50 x 10⁹/l platelet transfusion may be considered in an effort to control variceal bleeding.	Platelet count may show little increment following platelet transfusion in patients with splenomegaly.
• Baseline (i.e. pre-bleed) systolic BP is often lower than in non-cirrhotic patients.		

Table 14: *Replacing gastrointestinal blood loss in patients with chronic liver disease continued*

• Deficiency of coagulation factors is frequent.	Fresh frozen plasma is indicated only if there is documented coagulopathy. e.g. PTR >2.0.	Keep PTR <2.0 if possible. Complete correction is rarely possible with FFP due to the large volume.
• Giving red cells to try and raise Hb towards normal values may raise portal venous pressure, since blood volume is often increased. Over transfusion may contribute to rebleeding.		
• Provided blood volume is replaced and cardio-respiratory function previously adequate, a haemoglobin of 9 g/dl appears to be adequate.	Transfuse red cells to around 9 g/dl.	Coagulation factor concentrates have a risk of thrombo-genicity, in patients with liver disease. Use only with expert guidance.

Bleeding, especially if recurrent, is both intrinsically hazardous and is indicative of severe liver disease with a bad prognosis for the episode. A good outcome for the episode depends on overall management of infection, renal failure, ascites and encephalopathy.

Clinical applications of blood products

Warfarin (coumarin) anticoagulant overdose

Management should be guided by the principles in Table 15.

Table 15: *Management of warfarin overdose*

A Life threatening haemorrhage

Give 5 mg vitamin K by slow intravenous infusion and a prothrombin complex concentrate (PCC) containing Factors II, IX, X together with Factor VII (if available). The dose should be based on 50 iu Factor IX or Factor VII per kg body weight

If no concentrate is available, fresh frozen plasma should be infused (about 1 litre for an adult), but this may be less effective

B Less severe haemorrhage such as haematuria and epistaxis

Stop warfarin for 1 or more days. Vitamin K, 0.5 - 2.0 mg (iv slow infusion) will accelerate correction of abnormal clotting if this is clinically necessary

C Prothrombin time ratio expressed as INR of >4.5 without haemorrhage

Stop warfarin for one or two days: then review

D Unexpected bleeding at therapeutic levels of INR

Investigate the possibility of another cause, guided by the apparent site of bleeding

---

Thrombolytic therapy

Although bleeding is not a common complication of fibrinolytic therapy at normal doses, the risk is not predicted or reduced by laboratory monitoring. If rapid reversal of the fibrinolytic state is necessary because of serious bleeding, fresh frozen plasma will reverse the acquired deficiencies of Factor V and VIII:C; cryoprecipitate will raise a very low fibrinogen level. Antifibrinolytic agents should be used only if there is life-threatening bleeding. They may cause large clots at the site of bleeding, with severe clinical problems. They should not be used in intracranial or renal tract bleeding.

Cardiopulmonary bypass

Cardiopulmonary bypass usually impairs haemostasis due in part to its effect on platelet function. Especially in re-operations or in patients operated on for infective endocarditis, bleeding may be severe. Routine laboratory tests of coagulation do not accurately predict the clinical importance of the haemostatic defect. Platelet transfusion is indicated if there is microvascular bleeding or if the bleeding cannot be corrected surgically after the patient is off bypass and once heparinisation has been reversed with an adequate dose of protamine sulphate. Fresh frozen plasma helps to correct prolonged clotting times and may improve haemostasis, but the routine use of fresh frozen plasma or platelets at the end of bypass does not reduce transfusion requirements.

Aprotinin (Trasylol) can reduce transfusion requirements in specific situations such as valve surgery in patients with infective endocarditis but routine use is not advised for coronary artery or valve surgery in adults.

Congenital haemostatic disorders

Haemophilia

In the UK patients with Haemophilia A, Haemophilia B (Christmas disease), and von Willebrand's disease should be registered with and cared for by a Regional Haemophilia Centre. The Haemophilia Centre should be contacted when a patient with Haemophilia presents to a clinical unit. Detailed guidance on the products recommended for management of these patients is published by the UK Haemophilia Directors and regularly updated (*see Further reading*).

When a patient with haemophilia is seen away from a specialist centre it is important to get the best help available quickly (Table 16)

Clinical applications of blood products

4

Clinical applications of blood products   *61*

> **Table 16:** *Points to note in initial care of a bleeding Haemophilia patient*
>
> Identification: If the patient is unconscious, check if there is information carried on a bracelet or medallion. Contact the Haemophilia Centre for advice and inform the local haematologist.
>
> Products for treatment: Coagulation factor concentrates VIII and IX respectively are needed for Haemophilia A and B. The nearest supply may be in the patient's home provided for home therapy. In a real emergency and if clotting factor concentrates are unavailable, cryoprecipitate is the appropriate treatment for Haemophilia A and fresh frozen plasma is appropriate for Haemophilia B.
>
> Dosage: Factor VIII in a dose of 1 iu/Kg should give an immediate 2% rise in plasma Factor VIII. Factor IX (1 iu/Kg) should give an immediate 1% rise in Factor IX level.
>
> Monitoring: Clotting factor levels may be needed to assess response to treatment. Check with your local laboratory that these assays are available.

von Willebrand's Disease (vWD)

The assessment of treatment needs and response is not straightforward and needs measurement of both Factor VIII and von Willebrand's Factor. Some patients can be managed with desmopressin without the need for any blood product. If clotting factor replacement is needed a Factor VIII concentrate must be chosen that is effective for vWD. Cryoprecipitate was formerly the chosen replacement therapy but should now be used only if a virus-inactivated concentrate is not available.

Every effort must be made to obtain immediate specialist assistance in the management of these patients.

Transfusion in chronic anaemia

Nutritional replacement therapy with iron, vitamin B12 or folic acid or correction of the source of blood loss based on a correct diagnosis should be the treatment in most cases. Chronically anaemic patients are deficient in red cells but have a normal or increased blood volume. A rapid rise in haemoglobin is rarely required. In rare cases when red cell transfusion is felt to be needed, red cells (rather than whole blood) should be used to minimise the volume given. Patients who are elderly or who have cardiovascular disease or megaloblastic anaemia are most at risk of developing cardiac failure. Therefore red cells should be given slowly (4 hours per unit) at a time when the patient can be observed. A diuretic such as frusemide should be given if there is felt to be a risk of circulatory overload. *Do not add the diuretic to the blood component pack.*

Transfusion dependent anaemia

Regular red cell transfusion may be required for patients with myelodysplastic syndromes, chronic lymphocytic leukaemia, aplastic anaemia or malignant infiltration of the bone marrow.

Haemoglobinopathies

Patients with beta thalassaemia major or severe complications of sickle cell disease may need long term red cell support. These patients all require specialist investigation and management. Special precautions must be taken to reduce the risk of developing antibodies to red cells and white cells and the patient should be vaccinated against Hepatitis B and Hepatitis A. Accumulation of iron should be minimised by using a chelating agent (desferrioxamine).

In patients with thalassaemia the aim of a regular red cell transfusion regime is to suppress endogenous red cell production and keep the haemoglobin between 10.5 and 15.0 g/dl. In the other conditions mentioned above the need for transfusion is determined by the patient's clinical symptoms of anaemia.

If a patient is a potential candidate for bone marrow transplantation it is important to obtain expert advice before starting transfusion as special selection of blood products will be needed.

Anaemia in chronic renal failure

The treatment of choice is epoetin to maintain an adequate haemoglobin without the need for regular transfusion. Epoetin should be used according to the local hospital protocol.

Clinical applications of blood products

Bone marrow failure and transplantation

The treatment of malignant haematological disease or solid tumours often causes bone marrow suppression that requires transfusion support with platelets and/or red cells. In these patients transfusion may be complicated by graft-versus-host-disease (GvHD), cytomegalovirus (CMV) infection, or the development of antibodies to HLA antigens. The latter can cause non-haemolytic febrile transfusion reactions and may reduce the clinical effectiveness of platelet transfusions. Special precautions can help to minimise these problems.

Red cell transfusion

The principles are given on page 48. Patients should be tested periodically to detect the appearance of antibodies to red cells. Check again for red cell antibodies if there is a pyrexial reaction to red cells, an unexplained fall in haemoglobin or if the clinical response to red cell transfusion is less good than expected.

Platelet transfusion

A platelet transfusion regime should be set for the patient. The aim is to balance the risk of haemorrhage against the risks of repeated platelet transfusion (infection and alloimmunisation). The presence of clinical signs such as mucosal or retinal haemorrhage or purpura in a patient with a low platelet count generally indicate the need for platelet transfusion to control bleeding.

Most platelet transfusions are however given prophylactically and the policies of individual clinical teams differ. For stable afebrile patients, platelets are not usually given provided the count is above $10 \times 10^9/l$. If the patient has a fever and is suspected or known to have an infection, the threshold for platelet transfusion is usually $20 \times 10^9/l$. If the patient is stable platelet transfusion should be given to maintain platelet count: transfusion on alternate days is often sufficient. The adult dose of platelets is usually intended to contain at least 240×10^9 platelets. This can be provided either by pooling platelets prepared from 4-6 whole blood donations or by a single donor apheresis platelet unit.

Patients receiving intensive blood product support should be checked periodically for the development of antibodies to HLA Class I antigens especially if there are febrile reactions to platelet transfusions or if the increment in platelet count is less than expected. Poor increments are often seen if there is bleeding, infection or splenomegaly. If a poor platelet increment occurs in the presence of HLA Class I antibodies, the patient may benefit from receiving HLA matched or crossmatch-compatible platelets. However, about a third of refractory patients continue to show a poor response even if HLA matched platelets are given.

Refractoriness to platelet transfusion

Avoiding the development of antibodies to HLA antigens.
About half of all intensively transfused patients develop HLA Class I antibodies. In some this leads to febrile transfusion reactions and may accompany a poor response to platelet transfusion, often called refractoriness to platelets. A simple definition of refractoriness is that the patient's platelet count fails to rise by at least 10×10^9/litre the next morning after a platelet transfusion.

This simple measurement may help to predict the effectiveness of platelet transfusion in preventing clinically important bleeding.

Recently there has been much emphasis on avoiding the stimulation of HLA antibodies by the use of leucocyte depleted blood components. While this may be important there is still very little evidence that avoiding HLA alloimmunisation improves the clinical effectiveness of platelet transfusion. This remains a controversial subject. The practice of individual clinicians may continue to differ until the results of further clinical trials have been assessed.

To avoid alloimmunisation the patient should consistently receive, from the start of treatment, blood products that have a white cell content below 5×10^6 per dose. These are made either by plateletpheresis or by filtration of platelets or red cells with special filters. These filters can be used at the time of transfusion but this is less reliable than filtering the blood component under controlled laboratory conditions.

Clinical applications of blood products

Some units restrict the use of leucocyte depleted blood components to patients who experience repeated non-haemolytic febrile transfusion reactions.

All patients with aplastic anaemia who may later receive a bone marrow transplant should be given leucocyte depleted red cells and platelets. This is because HLA antibodies can reduce the chance of a successful 'take' of a bone marrow transplant.

Graft-versus-host-disease(GvHD): use of gamma-irradiated blood components.

Engraftment of viable lymphocytes transfused with whole blood, red cells or platelets can cause fatal GvHD in patients with severely depressed T-cell immunity e.g. after progenitor cell grafting. *This **must** be prevented by irradiation of all cellular blood components (25-30 Gy). Leucocyte depletion by presently available methods **does not** protect against GvHD.*

Cytomegalovirus(CMV) transmission.

Since CMV infection is an important cause of mortality following transplantation bone marrow or peripheral stem cell transplant recipients should receive CMV antibody negative cellular blood products, according to the CMV serological status of patient and donor as shown below. Fresh frozen plasma and cryoprecipitate have not been shown to transmit CMV. Patients who should receive CMV negative cellular components include

- CMV negative allograft recipients receiving a CMV negative graft

- CMV negative autograft recipients
- CMV negative acute leukaemia patients prior to transplant
- All new patients with haematological malignancy until their CMV status is known
- HIV positive patients who are CMV negative
- For some neonatal transfusions and intrauterine transfusion (page 95).

Since CMV is leucocyte-associated an alternative is to use leucocyte filtered cellular components.

Selection of ABO groups for transfusion of bone marrow allograft recipients.

If the ABO groups of donor and recipient are different the selection of the ABO group of cellular components to be transfused must be discussed with the hospital transfusion department.

Renal transplantation

In the past, 1-2 units of red cells were transfused to patients awaiting transplantation because this led to improved graft survival. Most specialists now consider that immunosuppression with cyclosporin makes this unnecessary. Anaemia is usually treated with epoetin. If red cells are administered they should be leucocyte depleted to avoid development of HLA antibodies and reduce any risk of CMV infection.

Heart, heart/lung and liver transplantation

Where both donor and recipient are CMV negative, CMV negative red cells and platelets should be used.

Liver transplant patients often have major abnormalities of coagulation and a low platelet count. Local protocols should define the pre-operative and intraoperative use of blood components. Steps often taken to minimise blood usage during surgery include the use of aprotinin, red cell salvage and continuous infusion of fresh frozen plasma during critical stages of the operation.

Intravenous immunoglobulin for immunological disorders

Immune cytopenias

Auto-immune thrombocytopenic purpura (AITP):

IVIgG in high doses has a role in the management of some patients but it is not a substitute for standard treatment including steroids and splenectomy. IVIgG produces an increase in the platelet count of varying duration in about 70% of patients but it does not alter the natural course of the disease. IVIgG may be useful:

- To assist management of acute bleeding
- To cover surgery or delivery in patients with AITP if the low platelet count causes risk of haemorrhage

A total dose of 1-2 g/kg divided over 1-5 days is usual in patients with chronic AITP; further occasional doses of 0.4 g/kg may help to maintain an adequate platelet count.

Clinical applications of blood products

Renal failure has occurred in elderly patients following administration of high dose intravenous immunoglobulin. Caution should be exercised in patients with pre-existing renal disease and in the elderly who may be more susceptible.

The use of high doses is associated with an increased rate and severity of adverse reactions and *the maximum dose of* 2g/kg *must not be exceeded in a single course of treatment.* In the elderly, a maximum daily dose of 0.4 g/kg may be safer.

Neonatal alloimmune thrombocytopenia (NAITP) See p73

Neonatal thrombocytopenia due to maternal AITP

Post-transfusion purpura

IVIgG has been used in all these conditions with variable results. In NAITP clinical trials of high dose IVIgG given to the mother have not confirmed earlier reports that this could prevent or reduce the severity of the disorder. IVIgG given to the neonate is effective in about 50% of NAITP cases and may be used with donor platelets which lack the antigen against which the maternal antibody is directed. In neonatal thrombocytopenia associated with maternal AITP, IV IgG is effective in some cases.

In all these conditions the initial dose should be 1-2 g/kg. Specialist advice is essential.

Immunoglobulin treatment in antibody deficiency states

Primary hypogammagobulinaemia

These patients have an inherited deficiency in antibody production. They need life-long replacement therapy to avoid or control the infectious complications of immune deficiency. Because intramuscular IgG is often poorly tolerated due to pain at the injection site (especially in children) it may be impossible to maintain levels of plasma IgG sufficient to prevent recurrent infection. The treatment of choice is regular administration of IVIgG. The standard dose is 0.2 g/kg body weight every 3 weeks but the dose may require to be increased or infusions given more frequently if recurrent infections persist. It is usual to aim to keep the plasma IgG level within the range of normal values. If IMIgG has to be used the conventional dose is 0.025-0.05 g/kg weekly.

Haematological malignancies

Some patients with chronic lymphatic leukaemia or myeloma are unable to make effective antibodies and suffer from recurrent severe infections due to gram positive encapsulated bacteria (e.g. Strep. pneumoniae, H. influenzae) that respond poorly to antibiotics. IVIgG at a dose of 0.2-0.4 g/kg every 3-4 weeks has been shown to reduce the frequency of episodes of these infections.

HIV

Some children with HIV who suffer from recurrent bacterial infections benefit from IVIgG, 0.2 g/kg body weight every 3 weeks. Episodes of infection, antibiotic use and hospitalisation can all be reduced.

Other indications for intravenous immunoglobulin

IVIgG is recommended for routine use in Kawasaki disease where a dose regime similar to that used in ITP is effective.

Treatment with IVIgG has been reported to be followed by clinical improvement in many other conditions including neuromuscular disorders that are thought to have an immunological basis. Treatment with IVIgG should generally be part of a clinical trial or may be justified as a last resort measure.

Intramuscular immunoglobulin for preventing infection

Normal Human Immunoglobulin (NHIG) and so called specific immunoglobulin products (that contain higher levels of antibody against specific organisms) are used, often together with active immunisation, to protect against infection. A summary of the products and their use is given in Table 17. Further information is given in the Handbook on Immunisation Against Infectious Disease, (see Further reading).

Table 17: *The use of immunoglobulin preparations for prevention of infection*

Infection	Indications	Preparations, vial content	Dose [Intramuscular]
Hepatitis A	Contacts and travellers requiring short term protection.	**Normal Human Immunoglobulin (NHIG) 250 mg and 750 mg**	Under 10 yr 250 mg 10 yr + over 500 mg

Hepatitis A vaccine may be preferable for regular travellers or a long stay. NHIG may interfere with development of immunity from live vaccines. Administer live vaccines if possible at least 3 weeks after immunoglobulin.

Measles	Children and adults with compromised immunity who come into contact with measles.	**NHIG 250 and 750 mg**	Under 1 yr 250 mg 1-2 yr 500 mg over 3 yr 750 mg

Immunoglobulin may interfere with development of active immunity from live virus vaccines. An interval of at least 3 months must elapse after an injection of immunoglobulin before subsequent MMR vaccination is attempted.

Rubella	Pregnant contact where termination is not an option	**NHIG 750 mg**	750 mg

Normal Immunoglobulin after exposure does not prevent infection and is not generally recommended for protection of pregnant women exposed to rubella. It may be used when termination of pregnancy would be unacceptable. In this case it should be given without awaiting reports on the woman's serological status. Serological follow-up is essential.

Tetanus	High risk injuries to non-immune subjects	**Tetanus Immunoglobulin 250 iu**	250 or 500 iu

Use together with active (toxoid) immunisation in tetanus prone wounds in the following: (i) unimmunised subjects, (ii) immunisation history unknown, (iii) over 10 years since last tetanus vaccine. Dose 250 iu but use 500 iu if more than 24 hours have elapsed since injury or if there is heavy contamination of the wound.

Tetanus	Clinical tetanus	**Intravenous Tetanus Immunoglobulin; 2,500 iu vials (available from SNBTS on a named patient basis)**	30-300 iu/kg

Table 17–Continued: *The use of immunoglobulin preparations for prevention of infection*

Infection	Indications	Preparations, vial content	Dose [Intramuscular]
Hepatitis B	Needle stab or mucosal exposure. Sexual exposure	**Hepatitis B Immunoglobulin (HBIG)** 500 iu **500 iu**	

Administer immunoglobulin as soon as possible after exposure with hepatitis B vaccine.

Infection	Indications	Preparations, vial content	Dose [Intramuscular]
Hepatitis B	Newborn babies of high risk mothers	**Hepatitis B Immunoglobulin 100 iu** 200 iu	

Administer immunoglobulin as soon as possible and within 48 hours after birth with hepatitis B vaccine.

Infection	Indications	Preparations, vial content	Dose [Intramuscular]
Varicella Zoster	Immuno-compromised adult or neonatat contacts.	**Varcella Zoster Immunoglobulin (VZIG) 250 mg and 500 mg vials** For SNBTS products and doses consult SNBTS product compendium *(Further Reading)*	0-5 yrs 250 mg 6-10 yrs 500 mg 11-14 yrs 750 mg 15+ yrs 1000 mg.

VZIG should be given to: *Immuno-suppressed patients* who within three months of the contact have been on high-dose steroids (e.g. 2mg/kg/day of prednisolone for more than a week).
Bone marrow transplant recipients.
Infants up to four weeks after birth:
- whose mothers develop chickenpox (but not zoster) in the period seven days before to one month after delivery
- in contact with chickenpox or zoster and whose mothers have no history of chickenpox or who on testing have no antibody
- in contact with chickenpox and who are born before 30 weeks of gestation or weighing less than 1 kg; they may not possess maternal antibody despite a positive history in the mother.

Pregnant contacts of chickenpox without a *definite* history of chickenpox should be tested for V-Z antibody before VZIG is given since about two- thirds of women have antibody despite a negative history of chickenpox. Those *without* antibody require VZIG.
HIV positive individuals with symptoms should be given VZIG after contact with chickenpox unless they are known to have V-Z antibodies.

Other Immunoglobulin Preparations
The following special preparations are available [from Regional Transfusion Centres in Scotland].
Normal Immunoglobulin for intravenous use, Measles Immunoglobulin, Tetanus Immunoglobulin 2,500 iu pack for intravenous administration in treatment of Tetanus, CMV Immunoglobulin.
All these products are supplied with package inserts and must be prescribed and given according to the manufacturers' instructions.

Clinical applications of blood products

Table 17–Continued: *The use of immunoglobulin preparations for prevention of infection*

Infection	Indications	Preparations, vial content	Dose [Intramuscular]
Rabies	Bite or mucous membrane exposure to potentially rabid animals	**Human Rabies Immunoglobulin 500 iu**	20 iu/kg

Rabies Immunoglobulin is used with rabies vaccine to provide rapid protection until the vaccine becomes effective. The recommended dose must not be exceeded and should be given at the same time as the vaccine. Half the dose should be infiltrated round the wound and the remainder given by deep intramuscular injection at a site separate from that used for rabies vaccine.

Sources of Supply

England and Wales	Normal Immunoglobulin: CDSC, Central Public Health Laboratory (CPHL) 0181 200 6868 and other Public Health Laboratories. Blood Products Laboratory 0181 953 6191
	Tetanus Immunoglobulin: Regional Transfusion Centres.
	Hepatitis B Immunoglobulin: Hepatitis Epidemiology Unit, CPHL and other Public Health Laboratories.
	Rabies Immunoglobulin: Virus Reference Laboratory, CPHL.
	Varicella Zoster Immunoglobulin: CDSC at CPHL.
Scotland	All immunoglobulin products are supplied through the Regional Transfusion Centres

Immunoglobulin products from commercial suppliers may be available through hospital pharmacies.

Transfusion of the newborn infant

Normal values

The blood volume is 80 ml/kg for full term infants and around 100 ml/kg for pre-term infants, depending on gestational age. The normal range of haemoglobin concentration in full-term infants is 14-20 g/dl. Platelet counts range from 150 to 400 × 10^9/l. The prothrombin time and thrombin time can be slightly prolonged in full-term infants; more marked prolongation of coagulation times is seen in the pre-term. The level of vitamin K-dependent coagulation factors in the neonate is about 50% of the normal adult value. Fibrinogen and other coagulation factors are in the normal adult range at birth.

Table 18: Normal ranges for term and preterm infants			
	Term*	Preterm* (<37 weeks)	Adult
Haemoglobin, g/dl	14-20	12.6-20	13-18
Platelets × 10⁹/l	150-400	150-400	150-400
PT (sec)	12-17	14-22	12-14
APTT (sec)	25-45	35-50	25-40
TT (sec)	12-16	14-18	12-14
Fibrinogen g/l	1.5-3.0	1.5-3.0	1.75-4.5

Normal values for preterm infants depend on gestation.
* These values are illustrative only: results from each laboratory must be related to the laboratory's own normal range.

Thrombocytopenia in neonates

There is an increased risk of haemorrhage in pre-term infants with moderate thrombocytopenia ($50\text{-}100 \times 10^9/l$) and in full-term infants with platelet counts less than $20\text{-}30 \times 10^9/l$. The risk is increased if there is sepsis or coagulopathy. One donation of recovered platelets should normally produce an acceptable platelet increment in children under 10 kg bodyweight. If the plasma volume of the platelet concentrate is excessive, the blood bank may be asked to remove plasma to a minimum volume of 10-15 ml per platelet concentrate. Neonates with thrombocytopenia associated with *maternal* autoimmune thombocytopenia (AITP) generally respond well to intravenous immunoglobulin (IVIgG) in a dose of 2 g/kg body weight. Platelet transfusions have no value in prophylaxis of this condition but may be useful if there is bleeding.

Neonatal alloimmune thrombocytopenia (NAITP)

This is a rare, serious condition and specialist advice is required. NAITP is caused by maternal IgG alloantibodies against a fetal platelet specific alloantigen. High dose IVIgG (2 g/kg body weight) given to the neonate is effective in about 50% of cases. However the treatment of choice is to give platelets lacking the HPA antigen. In the absence of suitable donor platelets, the mother's platelets may be used. They <u>must</u> be washed to remove the plasma which contains the platelet antibody and <u>must</u> be irradiated.

Haemolytic disease of the newborn (HDN)

What causes HDN?

Haemolytic disease of the newborn is caused by antibodies that are produced by the mother. These antibodies are IgG and can cross the placenta and destroy the baby's red cells.

In the most severe cases of HDN the fetus may die *in utero* or be born with severe anaemia that requires replacement of red cells by exchange transfusion. There may also be severe neurological damage after birth as a result of a high bilirubin level. Effective care of the affected pregnancy and of the newborn requires the skills of a specialist team.

The antibodies that cause HDN are directed against antigens on the baby's red cells that are inherited from the father and are absent in the mother. The mother may develop these antibodies if fetal red blood cells cross the placenta (feto-maternal haemorrhage) during pregnancy or delivery. They may also result from a previous red cell transfusion.

Antibody to the Rh D antigen is the most important cause of HDN. It only occurs in pregnancies in Rh D negative women where the father is Rh D positive. The frequency of HDN due to anti Rh D has been greatly reduced by the prophylactic use of Rh D immunoglobulin and also because family sizes have become smaller.

Although ABO incompatibility between mother and fetus is common, severe HDN due to IgG anti-A and anti-B antibodies is very rare in Caucasians in the UK. It is more common in some black populations. IgG antibodies against other blood group antigens (Rhc Rhe, RhC, RhE, Fy^a, K) occur in about 0.5% of pregnancies. If the fetus is positive for the antigen, the haemolysis may be severe.

Screening in pregnancy

All pregnant women should have their ABO and Rh D group determined when they book for antenatal care at 12-16 weeks. This identifies Rh D negative mothers; the mother's blood is also tested for any IgG antibodies to red cells that could cause HDN. If these are found, the father's red cell type should also be determined. If he is homozygous for the antigen concerned the fetus will be positive also; if he is heterozygous, there is a 50% chance that the fetus will be positive. If an antibody is detected at booking, it should be monitored throughout the pregnancy in case the level of antibody increases.

If no antibodies are detected at booking, the pregnant woman should have a further antibody check at 28-30 weeks gestation.

If anti-D or other antibodies are found during early pregnancy the level should be checked in accordance with local protocols and taking account of specialist advice.

Prevention of HDN - use of Rh D immunoglobulin (Anti-D)

This blood product is administered to the Rh D negative mother when there is a risk that fetal Rh D positive red cells may enter her circulation, usually due to a feto-maternal bleed. Anti-D prevents the mother from being immunised and starting to produce anti Rh D antibodies.

Anti-D should be given as soon as possible after delivery in a dose of 500 iu to a Rh D negative mother who has no Rh D antibodies and who has a Rh D positive infant. The prevention is less effective if Anti-D is given later, especially after 72 hours, but even if the correct time for the dose is missed, Anti-D should still be given as it may give some protection.

A 500 iu dose gives protection for feto-maternal haemorrhage of up to 4 ml red cells.

A Kleihauer test (which determines the number of fetal red cells in the mother's circulation) should be done as soon as possible after the baby is delivered when the dose of Anti-D is being given. If this shows that the feto-maternal bleed is larger than 4 ml, extra Anti-D must be given in a dose of 125 iu/1.0 ml of red cells. These larger bleeds often occur with interventions such as caesarian section, manual removal of the placenta, in twin pregnancy or after abdominal trauma.

Rh D immunoglobulin should also be given to the Rh D negative mother in other situations where she may be exposed to the red cells of her fetus. These situations are stillbirth, abortion (including therapeutic abortion), threatened abortion, ectopic pregnancy, amniocentesis, chorionic villus or fetal blood sampling, external cephalic version, abdominal trauma (e.g. seat belt injury) and antepartum haemorrhage.

Since mothers with some of these conditions may be seen in general practice or in hospital emergency departments rather than in the obstetric unit, it is important to be alert to the risk of sensitisation and to check the mother's Rh D type. In these situations Anti-D immunoglobulin should be given without waiting to determine the probable Rh D type of the father.

Up to 20 weeks gestation 250 iu should be given. Later 500 iu should be given and a Kleihauer screening test is advised. If there is repeated APH in pregnancy, the 500 iu dose should be repeated every 4-6 weeks. The level of Anti-D in the mother's blood can be monitored and should be kept above 0.25 iu/ml.

Rh D immunoglobulin should also be used to prevent immunisation if for any reason blood components containing Rh D positive red cells or organs from Rh D positive donors have to be given to a Rh D negative woman of child-bearing age or if Rh D positive blood is inadvertently transfused. The dose is calculated to remove the estimated amount of red cells transfused, as explained above.

Routine antenatal prophylaxis with anti-D. There is evidence that anti-D given in the 3rd trimester (500iu at 28 and 34 weeks) can further reduce the incidence of sensitisation from the present UK level of 1.5% to about 0.2%. This practice is being introduced in some units in the UK.

Failure to protect. It is important to note that some Rh D negative women still develop Anti-D because of failure to give Rh D immunoglobulin as above. Careful attention to the running of the preventive programme is the only way of avoiding a risk of damage to the mother's future infants.

Management of HDN

Because severe HDN is now rare women who are at risk of an affected pregnancy should have access to care in a unit that maintains specialist experience through regular management of these problems.

The condition of the fetus must be monitored throughout pregnancy as there may be a need for early delivery or intrauterine transfusion.

Affected neonates may be extremely ill and require specialist intensive therapy.

Clinical applications of blood products

Chapter 5

Adverse effects
of transfusion

Adverse effects of transfusion

Overview

Blood products, like other treatments can both benefit and do harm to the patient. Good clinical practice depends on understanding both the benefits that the treatment can provide for each patient and the risks that the treatment may carry for that patient. An essential part of the equation is to take account of the potential benefits and risks for the patient of NOT using a blood product or of using an alternative.

Where does responsibility rest for the various processes and decision elements that make up good transfusion therapy? Essentially, the *manufacturers* must ensure the safety of the product and *clinicians* must prescribe and use it correctly. There are additional important tasks for which the *hospital transfusion department* usually carries the main responsibility. Table 19 gives a framework for understanding these tasks and responsibilities and summarises aspects of safety that are often of concern to patients, parents or relatives. Tables 26 and 27 provide a summary of all the important adverse effects.

Reporting

From 1996 a UK confidential reporting system will operate for serious adverse reactions thought to be due to transfusion. The phone and fax details for reports are given on page 113.

Acute haemolytic or bacterial transfusion reactions

The features are summarised in Table 20.

It is important to monitor the patient for at least the first 15 minutes of the infusion of each unit of blood to detect the earliest clinical evidence of acute reactions due to incompatibility or bacterial contamination.

Incompatible transfused red cells react with the patient's own Anti-A or Anti-B antibodies or other alloantibodies to red cell antigens. This reaction can activate complement and cause disseminated intravascular coagulation (DIC). Infusion of ABO incompatible blood almost always arises from errors in labelling the sample tube or request form or from inadequate checks when a red cell transfusion is being given.

If red cells are by mistake administered to the wrong patient, (i.e. any patient other than the one for whom the red cells were supplied) the chances of ABO incompatibility are about 1 in 3. The reaction is usually most severe if Group A red cells are infused to a Group O patient. In a conscious patient even a few mls of ABO incompatible blood may cause symptoms within 1 or 2 minutes (Table 20). The patient becomes restless or distressed and may experience pain at the infusion site, flushing, abdominal, flank or substernal pain and breathlessness.

Table 19: Risks of transfusion treatment – an overview

Risk	Impact on Patients or Prospective Patients	Who is Responsible?	Impact on Health Care Providers
Virus infections.	• Fear of receiving blood. • Anxiety. • Need reassurance. • Want alternatives or no blood. • Actual risk is extremely small.	Manufacturer of blood products Prescribing clinician	Very substantial: Pressure for autologous tx, use of expensive drugs such as epoietin. Risk of legal claims. High cost of trying to achieve zero-risk in transfusion.
Accidents e.g. receiving the wrong blood.	• Some patients worry about this. • Actual risk small but…. • Possibly under recognised.	Clinical Team HTD*	Risk of legal claims. Medicolegal risk to individual clinicians.
Bacterial contamination of blood product.	• Patients assume there is no risk. • Very hazardous when it happens. • Actual risk small.	Manufacturer of blood products. Anyone involved in transport and storage of blood products.	Risk mainly to blood product manufacturer and HTD.
Complications due to red cell antibodies other than antiA + anti-B.	• Patients have little knowledge. • Occasionally hazardous • Actual risks due to reactions are very small but …. • Over caution can contribute to delays when transfusion is needed urgently	HTD should detect the antibodies and supply safe blood. Clinical team should keep (and read!) good patient records and warn the hospital transfusion department of possible problems.	
Over transfusion (circulatory overload).	• Patients have little knowledge. • No data about incidence. • Probably under diagnosed and under reported	Clinical team.	
Non febrile haemolytic transfusion reaction	• Regular recipients of red cell and platelets often very aware. • Distressing and unpleasant - not life-threatening. • In at least 2% of transfusions to regular recipients. • Probably under reported	Clinical team. HTD and sometimes blood products manufacture.	Cause of sub optimal patient care, delays for the patient, extra hospital costs.
Not transfusing when it is necessary	• Patients expect this would never happen (apart from Jehovah Witness). • If there is undue fear of viruses, reluctance to transfuse may put elderly and frail patients at risk.	Clinical Team	

*HTD - Hospital Transfusion Department

In an unconscious or anaesthetised patient hypotension and uncontrollable bleeding due to DIC may be the only signs of an incompatible transfusion. Oliguria is common and is often followed by acute renal failure.

Table 20: *Acute haemolytic transfusion reaction – recognition*

Signs and symptoms may occur after only 5-10 ml transfusion of incompatible blood so observe the patient carefully at the start of the transfusion of each blood unit.

If the patient has any of the following stop the transfusion and investigate.

Symptoms:
- Feeling of apprehension or "something wrong"
- Agitation
- Flushing
- Pain at venepuncture site
- Pain in abdomen, flank or chest

Signs:
- Fever
- Hypotension
- Generalised oozing from wounds or puncture sites
- Haemoglobinaemia
- Haemoglobinuria

Fever is often due to a cause other than acute haemolysis. As an isolated finding a rise of 1.5C above baseline temperature during transfusion should be investigated.

In unconscious patients only the signs will be evident.

If an acute haemolytic transfusion reaction is suspected, the transfusion must be stopped and urgent steps taken to confirm or exclude this possibility. The differential diagnosis must include infusion of bacterially contaminated blood.

Adverse effects of transfusion

Treatment is described in Table 21.

Table 21: *Acute haemolytic transfusion reaction – management*

Investigation	Treatment
1 Check again that the compatibility label of the blood unit corresponds with the patient's ID band, forms and case-notes.	1 Stop blood. Replace giving set. Keep IV open with sodium chloride 0.9%.
If a mistake is found tell the blood bank urgently since the unit of blood intended for your patient could be transfused to another patient.	2 Insert bladder catheter and monitor urine flow.
2 Take 40 ml of blood for	3 Give fluids to maintain urine output >1.5 ml/kg/hr.
• Haematology	4 If urine output <1.5 ml/kg/hr insert CVP line and give fluid challenges.
5 ml in EDTA tube - FBC, platelet count, direct antiglobulin test (DAT), plasma haemoglobin.	5 If urine output still <1.5 ml/kg/hr and CVP adequate then give frusemide 80-120 mg.
5 ml in dry tube - Repeat compatibility testing.	6 If no diuresis follows frusemide then give mannitol 20% 100ml IV.
10 ml in citrated tube - Coagulation screen (prothrombin time, APTT, fibrinogen).	7 If urine flow 2 hours after 20% mannitol and frusemide is <1.5 ml/kg/hr. *Seek expert advice - acute renal failure is likely.*
• Clinical chemistry	8 If bacterial contamination is suspected treat with broad spectrum intravenous antibiotics. *Seek expert advice.*
10 ml for urea or creatinine and electrolytes.	
• Blood cultures	9 If the patient's plasma potassium rises >6.0 mmol/l give 50 ml 50% glucose intravenous solution with 10 units of insulin IV. Follow with infusion of 10% glucose IV solution containing 10 units of insulin over 4 hours. Resonium A by nasogastric tube or rectally may be needed to control potassium.
3 Return blood pack(s) and giving set to the hospital transfusion department for bacteriology.	
4 Check urinalysis. Monitor urine output.	
5 Run an ECG and check for evidence of hyperkalaemia.	
6 Arrange for repeat coagulation screens and biochemistry 2-4 hourly.	10 If disseminated intravascular coagulation (DIC) develops give blood components guided by clinical state and coagulation screen results.
	11 If the patient needs further transfusion use rematched blood. There is no increased risk of a second haemolytic reaction.

Reactions due to red cell antibodies other than ABO

Haemolytic reactions can be caused by other red cell antibodies in the recipient's blood, including anti Rh D, Rh E, Rh c and K (Kell). Reactions due to anti RhD are rare since patients generally receive Rh D compatible red cells. Reactions due to these antibodies are usually less severe than those caused by ABO incompatibility since they do not activate complement. Destruction of transfused red cells ⊗ is mainly in the spleen or liver. The patient may experience fever, nausea and shivering. However, the Jk (Kidd) and Fy (Duffy) antigens do activate complement and can cause severe intravascular haemolysis leading to renal and cardiac failure. Jk antibodies are often very difficult to detect in pretransfusion samples.

A falling Hb or a rise in Hb that is less than expected after transfusion together with a rise in bilirubin and a positive direct antiglobulin test indicates that the transfused red cells are being destroyed.

Delayed haemolytic transfusion reactions (DHTR)

In patients who have previously been immunised to a red cell antigen during pregnancy or by transfusion the level of antibody to the blood group antigen may be so low that it cannot be detected in the pretransfusion sample. About 1% of parous women have red cell antibodies that are often undetectable by routine methods before transfusion. After transfusion of red cells bearing that antigen a rapid, secondary immune response raises the antibody level so that after a few days, transfused red cells bearing the relevant antigen may be rapidly destroyed. The signs of this *delayed haemolytic transfusion reaction* appear 5-10 days after transfusion with fever, falling haemoglobin, jaundice and haemoglobinuria. Clinically significant delayed haemolytic transfusion reactions are rare. Although DHTR is seldom fatal, it can cause further problems for a patient who is already seriously ill.

Adverse effects of transfusion

Non-haemolytic febrile transfusion reactions (NHFTR)

Fever or rigors during red cell or platelet transfusion affect 1-2% of recipients, mainly those who have been immunised to leucocyte antigens by pregnancy or previous transfusion. Antibodies in the patient's plasma react against transfused leucocytes in the blood component. The symptoms are shivering usually 30-60 minutes after the start of the transfusion, followed by fever. Most reactions can be managed by slowing or stopping the transfusion and giving an antipyretic e.g. paracetamol. (Table 22.) It is important to remember that the symptoms could be due to an acute haemolytic transfusion reaction or bacterially contaminated blood. Recurrent severe reactions in patients who require repeated transfusions of red cells or platelets may be prevented by the use of leucocyte depleted blood components. Initially buffy coat depleted red cells should be tried. Leucocyte depletion filters, which are much more expensive should be used if these other methods do not alleviate the reactions.

Allergic reactions

The symptoms are urticaria and itch within minutes of the transfusion. Symptoms usually subside if the transfusion is slowed and antihistamine is given (e.g. chlorpheniramine 10 mg by slow intravenous injection or intramuscular injection in patients who are not thrombocytopenic). The transfusion may be continued if there is no progression of symptoms after 30 minutes.

Chlorpheniramine (10 mg parenterally) should be given before transfusion when a patient has previously experienced repeated allergic reactions.

Table 22: *Prevention of acute transfusion reactions*

- Febrile non haemolytic transfusion reactions (FNHTR).

    If the patient has had 2 or more FNHTR try:

    Paracetamol 1g orally 1 hour before transfusion

    Paracetamol 1g orally 3 hours after start of red cell transfusion

    Slow transfusion (RCC 4 hours, platelets up to 2 hours)

    Keep the patient warm

    If the above measures fail, try:

    Filtered red cells or platelets

    Apheresis platelets

- Allergic reactions.

    If the patient has 1 severe or 2 minor allergic reactions:

    Chlorpheniramine 8 mg orally 30 minutes before transfusion.

- Anaphylaxis.

    Usually unpredictable.

    If the recipient is IgA deficient do not transfuse until you have obtained expert advice.

Anaphylaxis

This is a rare but life-threatening complication. Treatment is summarised in Table 23. It may occasionally be associated with antibodies against IgA in patients who have extremely low levels of IgA in their plasma. If this is the suspected cause the patient should if possible not be transfused. Special products will be needed and the hospital transfusion department must be consulted.

Table 23: *Treatment of anaphylactic reaction during transfusion*

- Stop the transfusion
- Maintain venous access with 0.9% saline
- Maintain airway and give oxygen
- Give adrenaline 0.5-1mg i.m., repeated every 10 minutes according to blood pressure and pulse until improvement occurs
- Give chlorpheniramine 10-20 mg by slow IV injection
- Give salbutamol by nebuliser
- Get expert advice. If in doubt get the duty anaesthetist.

Transfusion related acute lung injury (TRALI)

This form of acute respiratory distress may be under-recognised. The cause is usually donor plasma that contains antibodies against the patient's leucocytes. Transfusion is followed by a severe reaction with chills, fever, non productive cough and breathlessness. The chest x-ray shows numerous mainly perihilar nodules with infiltration of the lower lung fields. The implicated donors are almost always multiparous women and are found to have antibodies to white cells.

Reporting to the Hospital Transfusion Department is important so that an implicated donor can be removed from the panel. Treat as for Adult Respiratory Distress Syndrome from other causes.

Fluid overload

When too much fluid is transfused or the transfusion is too rapid, fluid overload can lead to systemic and pulmonary venous engorgement. Pulmonary oedema and acute respiratory failure may follow. Signs may include dyspnoea, tachycardia and hypotension. Standard medical treatment is a diuretic (e.g. frusemide 20mg IV initially) and oxygen. The transfusion should be stopped or slowed. Volume overload is a special risk with 20% Albumin solutions.

Patients with chronic anaemia are normovolaemic or hypervolaemic and may have signs of cardiac failure before any fluid is infused. If the patient must be transfused give red cells rather than whole blood with diuretic therapy if required. Each unit should be given slowly and the patient closely observed. Restricting transfusion to one unit in each 12 hour period should reduce the risk of fluid overload.

Late complications of transfusion

Iron overload

Transfusion dependent patients receiving red cells over a long period become overloaded with iron. Chelation therapy with desferrioxamine is used to minimise accumulation of iron.

Graft vs host disease (GvHD)

GvHD is a rare complication of transfusion caused by T-lymphocytes. Immunodeficient patients e.g. recipients of an allogeneic bone marrow transplant and fetuses receiving intrauterine transfusions are at special risk for this disease.

GvHD has also occurred in immunologically normal patients after transfusion of a relative's blood (see page 13). Transfusion associated GvHD is fatal in almost all cases. *Acute* GvHD begins 4-30 days after transfusion with high fever followed by a diffuse erythematous skin rash progressing to erythroderma and desquamation. Gastrointestinal and liver dysfunction occur and pancytopenia is common.

GvHD is prevented by gamma irradiation of cellular blood components to a dose of 25-30 Gy.

Immunosuppression

Blood transfusion alters the recipient's immune system in several ways. Two concerns are:

- Could tumour recurrence rates be increased? Prospective clinical trials have not shown a difference in the prognosis for transfused versus non transfused patients or for recipients of autologous as opposed to allogeneic blood.
- Does transfusion increase the risk of postoperative infection? So far clinical trials have failed to prove that this occurs but further studies are required.

Post transfusion purpura (PTP)

PTP is a rare but potentially lethal complication of transfusion of red cells or platelets, most often seen in female patients. It is caused by platelet-specific alloantibodies. Typically 5-9 days after transfusion the patient develops an extremely low platelet count with bleeding. Treatment is with high dose corticosteroids combined with high dose intravenous immunoglobulin. If platelet transfusion is unavoidable platelets that are compatible with the patient's antibody should be used. Expert advice is needed in managing PTP.

Infections that can be transmitted by transfusion

The perceptions of the risks of transfusion have been greatly influenced by HIV transmissions that occurred before today's safety testing procedures were available.

Blood donors, like anyone else, can occasionally carry an infectious agent, sometimes for a long period, without having any clinical signs or symptoms. For this reason the laboratory tests shown in Table 24 are performed on every blood donation. No part of the donation can be released until all these tests are known to be clear. Computer systems are used to ensure that no blood with a positive test slips through the net.

There is very good evidence that with the donor selection and testing procedures used in the UK the risk of infection is extremely small (Table 25). Blood products have become steadily safer over the years as previously unknown viruses have been identified and screening tests for them have been introduced. There has also been continuous improvement in the selection and testing of donors and in manufacturing processes. Inspection, regulation and licensing of the transfusion services by the Medicines Control Agency is an important contributing factor.

Table 24: *Infection Tests – Every donation is checked for:*
• Hepatitis B virus surface antigen (HBsAg)
• Hepatitis C virus antibody (HCV Ab)
• HIV 1 and 2 antibody (Anti HIV 1, Anti HIV 2)
• Treponema pallidum antibody

Adverse effects of transfusion

Figure 4. Decline in HBsAg positive blood donations in the UK 1972–1993.

HBsAg Positives per 1000,000 donations

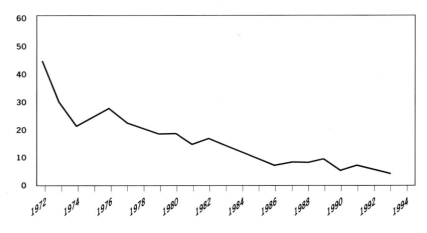

We can see something of how effective the systems are from the results on millions of donations that have been tested in pools of 10 to 20,000 before being used to make Factor VIII and other plasma fractions. (Fig 4)

The risk that a blood product may transmit an infectious agent depends on

● Prevalence and incidence in the community

● Combined effectiveness of the processes used to exclude and detect infected donors

● Virus inactivation

● Immune status of the recipient

● Number of individual donors contributing to each dose

Table 25 gives estimates of the risks of transfusion-transmitted virus infection.

Table 25: *Risks of transfusion-transmitted virus infections in the UK*

● Plasma fractions.
  Minimal risk of transmitting HIV, HTLV, HBV or HCV. Should non-enveloped viruses be present in donor plasma they may not be fully inactivated in all current products.

● Blood components.
  Not generally subjected to a virus inactivation step in production.

  HIV   Current estimate less than 1 per million blood components transfused. Only one reported incident due to HIV-screened blood in the UK since late 1985 when screening commenced.

  HBV   USA estimate: 1 per 200,000 components transfused in the USA. There is no UK estimate available.

  HCV   Current estimates for UK and USA less than 1 per 30,000 components transfused.

  HTLV I/II It is estimated that a maximum of 3 recipients per year in the UK have any lifetime risk of developing HTLV associated disease.

Hepatitis B

Figure 4 shows the steady reduction in the prevalence of Hepatitis B infection among blood in donors attending since the screening test first became available. Post transfusion Hepatitis B is exceedingly rare in the UK and no current figures for incidence are available.

Hepatitis C

Serological tests to detect Hepatitis C virus infection were introduced in 1991 and the tests have been progressively improved since then. The incidence of post transfusion hepatitis has reduced sharply: less than 1 in 30,000 blood components result in Hepatitis C infection and with the latest, more sensitive screening test the residual risk is being further reduced. The infection is usually asymptomatic and revealed only by disturbed liver enzyme tests. About half the affected patients develop chronic hepatitis that can lead after several years to severe liver damage.

Other Hepatitis viruses

Hepatitis A may very occasionally be transmitted by blood products. Further processes are being introduced to inactivate non-enveloped viruses such as Hepatitis A in plasma fractions. Hepatitis G may also be transmitted [see page 108].

HTLV (I and II)

HTLV I can cause neurological disorders and a rare form of adult T-cell leukaemia. There is usually a delay of many years between infection and development of illness. It is likely that only a small proportion of those infected become ill. HTLV I is transmissible by the transfusion of cellular blood components. The prevalence of infection is high in some parts of the world, notably Japan and the Caribbean. The link between HTLV II infection and disease is less clear, but infection is found in some intravenous drug users. Surveys in the UK indicate that the risk of HTLV related-disease following transfusion of blood is exceedingly low. Blood donors in the UK are not currently screened for HTLV I/II infection but the need for testing is regularly reviewed.

CMV

Approximately 50% of UK blood donors have antibody to CMV, but only a small proportion of antibody positive donations transmit the virus through transfusion. Transfusion transmitted CMV is of proven clinical importance in premature infants weighing less than 1200-1500g who are born to CMV antibody-negative mothers and in CMV antibody-negative bone marrow allograft recipients who receive CMV sero-negative grafts. Although the risk of clinical CMV infection is much smaller in recipients of autografts, some centres recommend that these patients also should receive CMV negative products. For these patients CMV safe blood components should be given. This is normally done by using donations that do not contain detectable antibody to CMV. An alternative is the use of leucocyte depleted blood components. Fresh frozen plasma and cryoprecipitate do not transmit CMV.

Human parvovirus B19

This non-enveloped virus may not be inactivated in all current plasma fractions. Processes are being developed to do this. There is evidence that HPV B19 infection is associated with bone marrow suppression affecting red cell production in occasional patients.

Treponemal infections

All donations are screened for serological evidence of Treponema pallidum infection. A further safeguard is that infectivity declines as blood is stored at 2-6C. Transfusion transmission is estimated to occur with a frequency of about 1 per 4 million in the USA. There appear to be no reports of transfusion transmission in the UK in recent years.

Chagas disease, caused by Treponema cruzii is transmissible by transfusion. This is an important problem in some South American countries where the infection is prevalent.

Adverse effects of transfusion

Other bacterial infections

Very rarely, bacterial contamination of a blood component occurs. This is a cause of very severe and often lethal transfusion reactions. In the UK, 16 incidents (9 fatalities) were identified during the 5 years to 1990, giving a rate of about 2 per million units transfused. Bacteria associated with severe septic reactions to red cell transfusion are usually cold-growing strains such as Pseudomonas fluorescens, an environmental contaminant or Yersinia enterocolitica, an organism that may enter a blood donor pack that is collected during an episode of asymptomatic bacteraemia. Skin contaminants such as staphylococci may proliferate in platelet concentrates stored at 20-22C and this is a factor limiting the safe storage life of platelet concentrates.

Malaria

Donor selection procedures are designed to exclude potentially infectious individuals from donating red cells for transfusion. Transfusion transmitted malaria occurs with a frequency of about 0.25 per million units collected in the USA. Comparable data for the UK are not available.

Table 26: *Acute complications of transfusion*

Problems	Cause	When? How often?	How dangerous?	Treatment Avoidance
Acute intravascular haemolysis of transfused red cells.	ABO incompatible transfusion. Group A donor into Group O recipient is worst.	Often during first few ml of infusion. About 1 in 500,000 red cell units transfused.	Mortality. 10% due to DIC and acute renal failure. Prevent: use safe documentation and checking systems for blood administration.	*Treat:* Page 84. *Avoid:* Page 32.
Infective shock.	Bacterial contamination of red cells or platelets with e.g. Pseudomonas, Yersinia, Staphylococci.	Usually during infusion of first 100 mls of the contaminated pack. 2 per million blood components transfused (UK).	Very high mortality	Treat: manage septicaemia. Fluids and intravenous antibiotics e.g. gentamicin plus ceftazidime.
Transfusion Related Acute Lung Injury. Non cardiogenic pulmonary oedema.	Donor plasma has antibody to patient leucocytes.	During or soon after transfusion. *Rare:* Greater risk if large volumes of donor plasma given e.g. whole blood or plasma exchange with donor plasma.	Life-threatening.	*Treat:* Respiratory support, diuretics and high dose steroids. *Avoid:* • Don't transfuse, especially plasma • Donor selection.
Non-Haemolytic Febrile Reactions (NHFTR) to transfusion of platelets and red cells.	Antibodies to transfused white cells. Usually from previous pregnancies or transfusions.	Within an hour or less. About 2% of all transfusion episodes. Mostly in patients who have had several previous transfusions.	Unpleasant, especially if the patient requires regular transfusions.	*Treat:* Paracetamol.* *Avoid:* Use leucocyte reduced or depleted cellular components.
Urticaria (allergic reaction).	Patient has antibodies that react with proteins in transfused blood components.		Unpleasant.	*Treat:* Temporarily stop infusion and give chlorpheniramine 10-20 mg iv. *Avoid:* Pre-medicate with chlorpheniramine 10-20mg iv before transfusion.

---

* A simple antipyretic is now thought to be as effective as chlorpheniramine and hydrocortisone. Paracetamol is preferred to aspirin since patients may be thrombocytopenic.

Table 27: *Delayed complications of transfusion*

Problems	Cause	When? How often?	How dangerous?	Treatment Avoidance
Delayed haemolysis of transfused red cells.	Patient has IgG antibodies to red cell antigens usually Rh c, E. C Kidd - Jka Duffy - Fya Kell - K	5-10 days after red cell transfusion. Less than 1/500 episodes of red cell transfusion.	Reduced survival of transfused red cells so transfusion may be less clinically effective. Consequences of haemolysis can complicate other conditions.	*Treat:* • No treatment for antibodies per se. • Once present, they are a problem for future red cell transfusions so: *Avoid:* • Write prominently in case notes. • Inform the hospital transfusion department when you next request red cells to transfuse the patient. • Good practice in pre-transfusion testing.
Development of antibodies to red cells in the patient's plasma (allo-immunisation)	Transfusion of red cells of a different phenotype from the patient. Also caused by fetal to maternal bleeding during pregnancy and child birth.	Days to weeks after transfusion. Anti RhD will develop in at least 75% of RhD negative patients transfused with a unit of RhD positive cells. Other red cell antigens stimulate antibodies much less frequently. 1-5% of previously transfused or parous patients have red cell antibodies. Antibodies are much more common in female patients.	Dangerous if the patient later receives a red cell transfusion. May cause haemolytic disease of the newborn.	*Treat:* • No treatment for antibodies per se. *Avoid:* *Avoid unnecessary transfusions - especially in premenopausal females.* • *Inform the hospital transfusion department when you next request red cells to transfuse the patient.* • *Good practice in pre-transfusion testing.*

Adverse effects of transfusion

Table 27 Continued: *Delayed complications of transfusion*

Problems	Cause	When? How often?	How dangerous	Treatment Avoidance
Development of antibodies that react with antigens of white cells or platelets.	Transfusion of blood cells of a different phenotype from the patient. Pregnancy.	About 40% of patients receiving platelet support for more than 2 weeks develop leucocyte and/or platelet antibodies. More likely if patient has a previous pregnancy.	Can cause unpleasant transfusion reactions (NHFTR). Patient antibodies to HLA antigens may contribute to a poor clinical response to platelet transfusion. Page 65. Post transfusion purpura - thrombocytopenia may be profound.	*Treat:* • No treatment for the antibodies per se. • If antibodies reduce clinical response to platelet transfusion, 'compatible' platelets may help (page). *Avoid:* • Use effectively leucocyte depleted red cells and platelets.
Iron overload.	One unit of red cells contains 250 mg of iron. It accumulates over a long course of red cell transfusion.	Clinical problems after several years of regular transfusion. Common in long term recipients of frequent red cell transfusion.	Liver damage and other problems are serious.	*Avoid:* • Planned transfusion regime. • Use chelating agent to increase iron excretion.

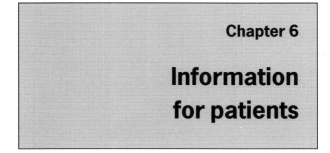

Chapter 6

Information
for patients

Information for patients

Principle

The Patients' Charter offers every patient the legal and ethical right before agreeing to treatment to receive adequate information about the risks and benefits of, and alternatives to, such treatment. The material risks of transfusion are sufficiently small that formal consent is not generally considered necessary. However, it is good clinical practice to provide adequate information to the patient and to make sure that it is understood. It is recommended that discussion with the patient should include the information in the following outline for a patient information leaflet.

An outline for a patient's guide

This leaflet explains why transfusion of blood is sometimes necessary. You may need transfusion as a planned part of your medical treatment or, if you are having an operation, it may be needed to replace blood loss. Although your consent to operation includes transfusion, it is important that you understand the reasons why blood transfusion might be advisable before you are asked to agree.

Transfusion of blood or individual constituents of it are given to correct abnormalities in your own blood system. This treatment is only advised when these abnormalities cannot be corrected by any other means. Common reasons for giving transfusion include:

1. **Loss of blood**
   An adult has about 10 pints of blood. Loss of small amounts, up to a pint of blood, for example during blood donation, causes no problems. Often loss of larger amounts does not need blood transfusion since other fluids, for example salt and water solution can be used to replace the loss. The loss of a larger amount of blood can be dangerous unless blood or a constituent of blood is given. For some operations, surgeons need to have blood available in case blood loss is more than expected.

2. **Anaemia**

   Anaemia means that the number of red cells in the blood is low. Anaemia often causes tiredness and breathlessness because the blood cannot carry enough oxygen to where it is needed in the body. There are many different causes for anaemia. Often treatment by drugs or vitamins is effective. If the anaemia does not respond or where rapid recovery is essential, blood transfusion may be the most effective form of treatment.

3. **Bleeding, blood clotting and other problems**

   Sometimes blood loses the ability to clot properly so that bleeding after injury continues for a long time. These problems can often be corrected by giving transfusions of blood products. These are usually purified clotting substances (for example the substance that haemophiliacs lack) or cells known as platelets that can be extracted from blood donations.

How does your doctor decide what to advise?

Your doctor has to decide when transfusion is the best remedy for the problem you have. Alternative treatment may be available and your doctor will decide whether these can be used instead. Blood transfusion treatment like other forms of treatment including medicines carries a very small risk of harmful effects. Doctors weigh these potential risks very carefully against the benefits of transfusion.

What are the risks?

Millions of transfusions, saving many lives, are given every year in the United Kingdom. The vast majority of these cause no harmful effects. HIV infection (the virus that causes AIDS) is perhaps the best known risk but the chance of this in the United Kingdom is less than one in a million. This safety is the result of very stringent measures taken by the Blood Transfusion Service to ensure the safety of the blood supply. Hepatitis (jaundice) is another possible complication. Every blood donation is tested for the viruses that cause hepatitis and AIDS.

Clotting factors and other blood protein products undergo virus killing processes that further reduce the risk of transmitted infection.

Other temporary side effects such as feverish reactions may occur. These are minimised by careful selection of blood in the hospital transfusion laboratory. They are usually insignificant compared with the expected benefit of transfusion.

Can I use my own blood for transfusion instead?

In some circumstances this is possible and sometimes it may be recommended. Your doctor will advise you about whether this would be useful in your own individual circumstances.

The Blood Transfusion Service in the United Kingdom is fortunate in having the support of very large numbers of voluntary blood donors whose only reward is the knowledge that they are giving blood for the benefit of others. For this reason blood transfusion in the United Kingdom is recognised to be among the safest in the world.

Sources of information

Further reading

Albumin

McClelland, D.B.L. ABC of transfusion.. Human albumin solutions. *Br med.J.* 1990, **300,** 35–37.

Plasma substitutes: the choice during surgery and intensive care. *Drug Ther. Bull.* 1987, **25,** 37–39.

Autologous Transfusion

British Committee for Standards in Haematology, Guidelines for Autologous Transfusion I. Pre-operative autologous donation. *Transfusion Med.* 1993, **3,** 307–316.

Cardiac Surgery

Goodnough, L.T., Johnston, M.F.M., Ramsey, G., Sayers, M.H., Eisenstadt, R.S., Anderson, K.C., et el. Guidelines for transfusion support in patients undergoing coronary artery bypass grafting. *Ann. thorac. Surg.* 1990, **50,** 675–683.

Spence, R.K., Alexander, J.B., DelRossi, A.J., Cernaianu, A.D., Cilley, J., Jr, Pello, M.J., et al. Transfusion guidelines for cardiovascular surgery:lessons learned from operations in Jehovah's Witnesses. *J. vasc., Surg.* 1992, **16,** 825–831.

Collection and Production of Blood Components

UKBTS–NIBSC Liaison Group. *Guidelines for the Blood Transfusion Service,* 2nd Edition. London: HMSO, 1993 (ISBN 0 11 321560 6).

Erythropoietin

MacDougall, I.C., Hutton, R.D., Cavill, I., Coles, G.A., and Williams, J.D. Treating renal anaemia with recombinant human erythropoietin: practical guidelines and a clinical algorithm. *Br. med. J.* 1990, **300,** 655–659.

General

McClelland, D.B.L. (Editor) *Optimal use of donor blood.* Report of a working party set up by the Clinical Resource and Audit group. London: HMSO, 1995 (ISBN 0 7480 2910 9).

Contreras, M. (Editor) *ABC of Transfusion Medicine,* London: British Medical Journal, 1990 (ISBN 0 7279 0288 1).

UK Regional Haemophilia Centre Directors Committee. Recommendations on choice of therapeutic products for the treatment of patients with haemophilia A, haemophilia B and von Willebrand's disease. *Blood Coagul. Fibrinolysis,* 1992, **3,** 205–214.

Wood, K. (Editor) *Standard Haematology Practice/2.* Oxford: Blackwell Science, 1994 (ISBN 0 632 03739 3).

Haemostasis and Thrombosis

British Committee for Standards in Haematology. Guidelines on oral anticoagulation: second edition *J.clin. Pathol.,* 1990, **43,** 177–183.

Immunoglobulins

Intravenous immunoglobulin: prevention and treatment of disease. NIH Consensus Conference. *JAMA,* 1990, **264,** 3189–3193.

Joint Committee on Vaccination and Immunisation. *Immunisation against infectious disease.* London: HMSO, 1992 (ISBN 0 11 321515 0).

New perspectives on the use of intravenous immune globulin. *Clin. exp. Immunol.* 1994, **97,** (Suppl. 1), 1–83.

Recommendations for off-label use of intravenously adminstered immunoglobulin preparations. Consensus statement. *JAMA,* 1995, **273,** 1865–1870.

Irradiation of Blood Components

British Committee for Standards in Haemotology. Guidelines on gamma irradiation of blood components for the prevention of transfusion-associated graft-versus-host disease. 1996 (in press).

Leucocyte Depleted Components

Royal College of Physicians of Edinburgh. Report of Consensus Conference on Leucocyte Depletion of Blood and Blood Components. 18–19 March 1993.

Massive Blood Loss

British Committee for Standards in Haematology. Transfusion for massive blood loss, in Roberts, B. (Editor) *Standard Haematology Practice.* Oxford: Blackwell Scientific Publications 1991, pp. 198–206 (ISBN 0 632 02623 5).

Neonatal and Paediatric Transfusion

Sacher, R.A., Luban, N.L.C., and Strauss, R.C. Current practice and guidelines for the transfusion of cellular blood components in the newborn. *Transfusion Med. Rev.* 1989, **3**, 39–54.

British Committee for Standards in Haematology. Guidelines for administration of blood products: transfusion of infants and neonates. *Transfusion Med.* 1994, **4**, 63–69.

Obstetric Haemorrhage

Report on confidential enquires into maternal deaths in the United Kingdom 1988–1990. London: HMSO, 1994 (ISBN 0 11 321691 2).

Plasma

British Committee for Standards in Haemotology. Guidelines for the use of fresh frozen plasma. *Transfusion Med.* 1992, **2**, 57–63.

Platelets

British Committee for Standards in Haematology. Guidelines for platelet transfusions. *Transfusion Med.* 1992, **2**, 311–318.

Prevention of Haemolytic Disease of the New Born

Lee, D. (National Blood Transfusion Service Immunoglobulin Working Party) Anti-D immunoglobulin [Editorial]. *Prescribers' J.* 1991, **31**, 135–136.

Procedures and Documentation

British Committee for Standards in Haematology. Guidelines on hospital blood bank documentation and procedures. *Clin. lab. Haematol.* 1990, **12**, 209–220.

Red Cells

Perioperative Red Blood Cell Transfusion. Consensus Conference. *JAMA* 1988, **260**, 2700–2703.

Flanagan, P. Red cell transfusions including autologous transfusion. *Prescribers' J.* 1992, **32**, 15–21.

American College of Physicians. Practice strategies for elective red blood cell transfusion. *Ann. intern Med.* 1992, **116**, 403–406.

Welch, H.G., Meehan, K.R., and Goodnough, L.T. Prudent strategies for elective red blood cell transfusion. *Ann. intern Med.* 1992, **116,** 393–402.

Consensus statement on red cell transfusion. Proceedings of a Consensus Conference held by the Royal College of Physicians of Edinburgh, 9–10 May 1994. *Br. J. Anaesth.* 1994, **73,** 857–859.

Accessing the evidence-base for this handbook.

The editorial team have agreed to assemble a 'hypertext' version to help to access sources of evidence that underlie the statements in this book.

Readers who are interested in helping us to develop this product or in using it once it is available are invited to contact the editor.

Hepatitis G

Hepatitis G has recently been identified. It can only be detected by gene amplification technologies and no test for donor screening is available. It is not known whether Hepatitis G can cause serious disease: at present it appears that it may not. The agent has strong similarities to Hepatitis C virus and is probably inactivated by existing procedures in plasma fraction manufacture.

Table 28: *Telephone and Fax numbers of regional transfusion centres*

	Tel No.	Fax No.
National Blood Authority (HQ)	01923-212121	01923-211031
Scottish National Blood Transfusion (HQ)	0131-664-2317	0131-658-1639
Newcastle Blood Transfusion Centre (Northern)	0191-261-1711	0191-232-4554
Leeds Blood Transfusion Centre (Yorkshire)	01132-645091/2/3	01132-603925
Sheffield Blood Transfusion Centre (Trent)	01142-424242	01142-435083
Cambridge Blood Transfusion Centre (East Anglia)	01223-245921	01223-411618
North London Blood Transfusion Centre **(Colindale)**	0181-200-7777	0181-200-3994
Essex Blood Transfusion Centre **(Brentwood)**	01277-223545	01277-225662
South Thames Blood Transfusion Centre **(Tooting)**	0181-672-8501/7	0181-767-4462
Southampton Blood Transfusion Centre (Wessex)	01793-776441	01703-704067
Oxford Blood Transfusion Centre	01865-741188	01865-741343
Bristol Blood Transfusion Centre (South West)	01179-507777	01179-592552
Birmingham Blood Transfusion Centre (West Midlands)	0121-414-1155	0121-414-1308
Liverpool Blood Transfusion Centre (Mersey)	0151-709-7272	0151-709-0392
Manchester Blood Transfusion Centre (North West)	0161-273-7181	0161-274-3941
Lancaster Blood Transfusion Centre (North West)	01524-63456	01524-62602
Cardiff Blood Transfusion Centre (Wales)	01222-890302	01222-890825
Belfast Blood Transfusion Centre (Northern Ireland)	01232-321414	01232-439017
Aberdeen Blood Transfusion Centre (North East Scotland)	01224-685685	01224-662200
Dundee Blood Transfusion Centre (East Scotland)	01382-645166	01382-641188
Edinburgh Blood Transfusion Centre (South East Scotland)	0131-536-5300	0131-536-5352
Glasgow & West of Scotland Blood Transfusion Centre	01698-373315/8	01698-356770
North of Scotland Blood Transfusion Centre **(Inverness)**	01463-704212/3	01463-237020
Dublin Blood Transfusion Centre	00-353-1-603333	00-353-16-603419
Cork Blood Transfusion Centre	00-353-21-968799	00-353-21-313014
Central Public Health Laboratory (CPHL)	0181-200-6868	
Serious Hazards of Transfusion: Reports to: Dr. Elizabeth Love	0161-273-7181	0161-236-6904 [confidential fax]

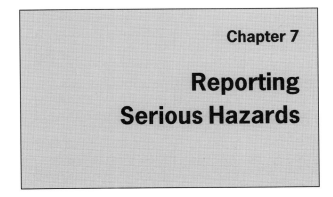

Chapter 7

Reporting
Serious Hazards

UK Project on Reporting Serious Hazards of Transfusion

The Serious Hazards of Transfusion (SHOT) Group, with representatives from the UK Colleges of Physicians, Surgeons, Obstetricians, Nursing, Institute of Biomedical Scientists, Transfusion Services and other relevant professional bodies, plans to start a voluntary central reporting system for serious adverse events following transfusion of blood or labile blood components (Fresh Frozen Plasma, Platelets, Cryoprecipitate, Granulocytes).

It is hoped that this confidential reporting system will lead to an increased awareness of the frequency of adverse events in this setting and factors contributing to their occurrence. Analysis of these reports may lead to recommendations for changes in practice which will improve transfusion safety.

This reporting system will not replace the current systems in place for reporting *infectious* complications of transfusion which should be reported to your local Transfusion Centre as soon as this diagnosis is suspected. Neither is it intended to replace mechanisms which already exist for advice and investigation of any adverse event by your local Transfusion Centre.

Adverse events secondary to the administration of *fractionated* plasma products (e.g. Intravenous Immunoglobulin) should be reported to the Committee for Safety of Medicines using the current Yellow Card System.

The SHOT reporting system is planned to commence in 1996. A short, initial report form will be widely distributed prior to commencement of the scheme and further information will be circulated at that time.

On page 113 you will find an "aide-memoire" to the most frequently encountered adverse events and the relevant diagnostic tests. Your local Haematologist will be able to give more detailed advice on management and investigation.

Medical Co-ordinator of the UK Project on Reporting of Serious Hazards of Transfusion

Dr Elizabeth Love, Consultant Haematologist, Manchester Blood Centre, Plymouth Grove, Manchester M13 9LL
[Telephone 0161 273 7181 Confidential Fax 0161 236 6904].

SERIOUS HAZARDS OF TRANSFUSION (SHOT)

Summary of Key Features and Diagnostic Tests for Adverse Events

Problem		Typical features	Diagnostic Tests
1.	**Incorrect Blood or component transfused**		
	ABO incompatible	May be none—or major collapse as for 2	Check identity and group of patient and unit [inc. Rh(D)]. May have +ve DAT
	ABO compatible	May be none. As for 2 if patient has atypical red cell alloantibodies	Check identity and group of patient and unit [inc. Rh(D)]. May have +ve DAT
2.	**Major acute or delayed transfusion reaction**		
	Acute haemolytic transfusion reaction	Dyspnoea, chest pain, fever, chills, ↓BP, ↓urine output, DIC	Haemo-globinaemia /uria, ↓Hb, +ve DAT, serological incompatibility, spherocytes on blood film
	Delayed haemolytic transfusion reaction	Unexplained fall in Hb. Jaundice, dark urine	Urobilinogen in urine, ↑serum bilirubin, +ve DAT, spherocytes, +ve antibody screen
	Anaphylaxis	↓BP, dyspnoea, ±rash	Occasionally severe IgA deficiency with anti-IgA

Reporting Serious Hazards

Summary of Key Features and Diagnostic Tests for Adverse Events

Problem	Typical features	Diagnostic Tests
3. **Transfusion-Associated Graft-Versus-Host Disease (TA-GVHD)**	Progression of fever, rash, ↑liver enzymes, diarrhoea, pancytopenia (1–6 weeks post transfusion)	Skin biopsy +cytogenetic or HLA analysis. DNA analysis (e.g. RFLP, minisatellite probes) to establish presence of third party lymphocytes
4. **Transfusion-Related Acute Lung Injury (TRALI)**	Acute respiratory distress (non cardiogenic) hypoxia, bilateral pulmonary infiltrates	Anti-leucocyte antibodies in donor or recipient
5. **Post-Transfusion Purpura (PTP)**	Immune-mediated thrombocytopenia arising 5–12 days post-transfusion	HPA type patient. HPA antibodies (usually HPA-1a negative with anti-HPA-1a)
6. **Reaction to a bacterially contaminated component**	Rapid onset of circulatory collapse, fever	**REFER TO REGIONAL TRANSFUSION CENTRE URGENTLY**
7. **Post transfusion viral infection**	Depends on virus. e.g. Jaundice, malaise, rash. Weeks to month post transfusion	**REFER TO REGIONAL TRANSFUSION CENTRE URGENTLY**
8. **Other**	Any other severe adverse reaction associated with transfusion of a blood component	

Index

Printed in the United Kingdom for HMSO   Dd301683 6/96 C800 G569570 10170